The Big BOOK for LiTTLeS

The BiG BOOK *for* LiTTLeS

Tips & Tricks for Age Players & Their Partners

by Penny Barber

First Edition

Pennyroyal Press

San Francisco

For bulk orders email mr.samsolo@gmail.com.

TABLE OF CONTENTS

THank you

A lot of people helped me put this book together. M. D. L., thank you for always being available when I've needed an editor and for your gentle criticism. Mako Allen, thank you so much for your suggestions, insight, correction, time, and expertise.

Sam Solo, my little darling, how could I accomplish anything without my right hand? You've supported me figuratively and literally, pulled me up when I was down. When I needed you to be good at a something, you developed the skill. When I needed to rant, you listened patiently. I will never be able to repay what you have given so freely. I am proud to see my collar on your neck.

And thank you to my clients, fans, and other supporters. God knows what I'd be doing with my life without you, but it certainly wouldn't be this cool and interesting. Thank you for sharing my fantasies!

Foreword

by Mako Allen

There's a story I've told for years about an awkward interaction an ex of mine and I had with another age playing couple. We had met the couple at one of the quarterly munches we held in the Inner Harbor in Baltimore. The man was an adult baby, and had been for a very long time. His partner was experienced in BDSM and kink, but new to being her boy's Mommy.

We passed a lovely afternoon with them and many other folks, and after the munch was over, spent even more time with the couple. They were charming and fun. Eventually, we had them back to our house for dinner, socializing, and possibly other things.

At a certain point, the boy and I were talking in the living room as my ex and his Mommy had their own conversation in the kitchen. He fussed, almost delightedly, at how he really needed his wet diaper changed, and confided in me about how very much he was looking forward to the pair of us being seen to by the pair of them. I started to tell him that that's not how things work, to not hold onto expectations, to be present, quiet, and respectful, and allow things to unfold organically without being pushy.

It went in one ear and out the other.

When our Mommies came back into the living room he turned to them and said, demanded really, "Okay, do the age play now."

I cringed inside. My Mommy and I gave one another a knowing, pained look, and the smallest of awkward smiles.

His Mommy didn't take it so well. She was genuinely ashamed of his behavior which, to be honest, had been terrible. He was demanding, selfish, and entitled.

After he apologized and they left, my Mommy told me, "I'm so glad you know better." I was glad, too, and I was glad to hear that Penny Barber was writing this book, and asked me to write the foreword for it.

"Doing the age play" is actually not a simple thing. I'm 45 years old, and have known I was an age player since before I knew the term. I can recall being in my early teens and having fantasies about being diapered and getting spanked. I was fortunate enough to stumble across some highly instructive self-help material. (A particular copy o f *Penthouse Variations* was especially helpful.) But for years I labored to come to a place of understanding about these things I wanted. I thought that perhaps something might be very wrong with me.

Just after I graduated college, I made the decision to embrace this part of myself. I went to go see a therapist to get myself a "checkup from the neck up." Turns out, I was just fine, and that there's nothing wrong with being kinky in general, or with being an age player in particular.

I spent the next two decades living the age play life I had always wanted, but never before truly allowed myself. Along the way I made plenty of mistakes, but learned a bunch too. At one point I de - cided that it wasn't enough for me to live a fulfilled life as an age player--I wanted to help others to come to that place of self-love and self-knowledge that I had sort of stumbled into, almost by accident.

I started going on podcasts, teaching classes at kink events, writing fiction about being an age player and eventually, along with my part- ner Spacey and his wife, Mae, started my own podcast, The Big Little Podcast (biglittlepodcast.com).

Somewhere in all this, I first learned about Penny Barber.

Penny's something of a legend amongst age players. She's an incredibly well-known adult film star, one of the very first to openly specialize in age play and diaper fetishes. She's also a sex worker, a professional dominatrix who specializes in diaper discipline, among other things.

As I got to know her I saw that she has that same drive that I do. Getting her own ass spanked and diapered isn't enough for her. She wants to help others to figure themselves out and get what they need.

Her work is profoundly good. It rings true. When she diapers and spanks someone else, you can tell that she genuinely is aroused by it, and understands what it means to play like that. When someone else is diapering her, you can see how deeply it affects her emotionally and sexually. That's because she's an age player, through and through. She knows how to "do the age play."

That's why this book is such a good thing. She lays it all out for you, as a fellow Little. She tells you how to figure out what speaks to you, what you want and need. She tells you how to tell a partner about it.

And this is not a simple thing. What if you're Little, but want to be dominant? Can you even do that? (Spoiler, you totally can.)

This book is filled with common sense guidance that is valuable to age players at every level of experience. Think of it as *Being Little for Dummies*--except that the fact that you're reading this book shows that you're no dummy at all. This book covers an incredibly wide gamut of topics about the many and various ways one might indeed "do the age play."

Take my advice, listen to her. Penny knows what she's talking about.

I hope you enjoy reading this book as much as I have, and learn a little something, too.

Mako Allen
July 2, 2016

introduction

Almost immediately upon releasing *The Age Play and Diaper Fetish Handbook*, I noticed ways in which it could be improved and I was very open to feedback from others. *The Big Book for Littles* started as a second edition of the *Handbook*, but as the Littles community continued to develop, I began to imagine the project as a sort of community effort. Alas, getting age players to submit content proved to be prohibitively difficult and that idea was scrapped, too-- at least for now. Perhaps it will work out in the future!

I ended up starting over entirely. As a result, *The Big Book for Littles* is more like a companion piece to *The Age Play and Diaper Fetish Handbook*. Because I'm so heavily involved in age play, this book, like the one before it, is largely influenced by my own experiences. I've personally done just about everything mentioned within-- many times, if it was really good. Hence, the writing is almost auto-biographical, and I can't imagine writing something so close to my heart in any other way.

With my first book, I tried to find a publisher, but was turned down left and right by people who seemed to think that there wasn't enough of a market to support a book about age play and--gasp!--diaper fetishism. Luckily, they were wrong and the book did well! I'm glad that I stuck it out. This time around, I decided to go straight to self-publishing.

A note on the evolution of my writing: I penned the *Handbook* in a sort of old-fashioned style, probably as a result of reading too many Aristasia novels. In an attempt to be gender-neutral, but still keeping with widely accepted grammar rules, I used the indefinite pronoun "one". Unfortunately this proved to be confusing, even to self-proclaimed grammar nerds. Hence, in this book, I've just written in my own vernacular and used the pronouns "they" and "you". It's equally inclusive and less confusing.

This is one of those books that is best read in pieces and not just straight through. Think of it as a reference rather than a curriculum. Skip around and look things up as they become relevant to you or as they pique your curiosity.

I hope that you get what you're looking for out of this piece, that it helps make your age play more fulfilling and enjoyable. I mean to remain open to criticism and make my next work even better!

Penny Barber
January 13, 2016

Little Space

Defining Age Play

While there are pre-written definitions out there, I recommend creating a definition for age play that highlights what *you* do, a description of *your* Little self. You can start with something simple and universal, like: *Age play is roleplaying, where people behave and perhaps are treated as though they were a different age than they actually are. Usually, it's a younger age, but it can be older as well.*
Then you can build up to more meaningful specifics. This can help
strengthen your age play identity.

Which activities qualify as age play vary from person to person, and,
unlike a lot of other hobbies, age play doesn't just mean engaging in
certain actions, but being in a certain mindset or headspace, often

called "Little space". For example, if I'm crocheting, I'm crocheting. I don't have to be feeling a certain way because it's just a physical act. However, if I'm coloring in a coloring book, I may or may not be age playing, based on whether or not I'm in Little space as I color. The nuances of that certain Little space are unique to each individual, but getting there is what age play is all about for many people.

Of course tacking down definitions for subcultures--and subcultures within subcultures--often alienates their members. For example, if one defines domestic discipline as non-sexual BDSM, BDSM practitioners who do not have sex as part of their play or perhaps at all will firmly state that they do not practice domestic discipline. Domestic discipline players who *do* engage in sexual play or who define discipline as sex will likewise feel ostracized and even outraged.

As you move through the world, you may encounter someone who sees the age play community as a safe haven for their antisocial, predatory behavior. Age play is not inherently abusive and is completely distinct from pedophilia. If you are unlucky enough to encounter one of these people, make it clear that they are *not* welcome in your community or around you personally. Report them to community leaders or moderators if possible, then move on.

Remember to log distressing online conversations with screen captures and save them. Before making a report to anyone, you need to be able to prove that this person was behaving inappropriately so that law enforcement or site administrators can begin investigating. Never save inappropriate or illegal images, as this practice will incriminate *you*, not just the person who posted or sent them. If you have a concerning in-person interaction with one of these people, you can always write down the details or record yourself talking about it in order to create a sort of record. Hopefully you'll never have to do any of this, but it's good to know how to handle these situations in advance.

If, when trying to introduce your Little self to a partner, they mistake age play for pedophilia, try not to freak out. I don't understand why this confusion keeps coming up, since the age play that I encounter is in groups which are strictly for those of us over the age of 18. But it does happen, so it's best to be prepared.

Explain again that you are an adult and that you're only interested in adults, that you understand the difference between a roleplay power dynamic and child abuse and hope that your partner does, too. Remind them that they don't have to do anything that makes them uncomfortable, and that you were just hoping to share a little more of yourself with them.

Don't overwhelm your partner. Give them time to think about it and ask you questions. You can give your partner some time alone to let the information sink in if that's what they need. You might want to mention that, if they choose to do some research on age play on their own, the things that they look up online may not apply to you or may simply be wrong.

If you want a textbook definition of age play, the closest would probably be the medical definition of paraphilic infantilism. Wikipedia offers the following definition for the entry *paraphilic infantilism*. While it's technically correct (at least for some sexual, infantilistic age players), it's also somewhat outdated and a little disappointing, but it's similar to definitions from various medical texts.

> *A* sexual fetish *that involves* role-playing *a regression to an infant-like state. Behaviors may include drinking from a bottle or wearing diapers. Individuals may engage in gentle and nurturing experiences (an adult who only engages in infantilistic play is known as an adult baby) or be attracted to masochistic, coercive, punishing or humiliating experiences. ... When wearing diapers, infantilists may urinate or defecate in them.* [1]

Other medical terms relevant to age play include:

Adult baby syndrome This term was coined in a 2002 episode of *ER*.[2] It was adopted by the medical community in 2003 in an article in *the American Journal of Psychiatry* by Drs. Pate and Gabbard.[3] They described the syndrome according to its manifestation in a man who engaged in solo and isolating age regression roleplay when not at work. This play sometimes included masturbation in diapers, which he used for both urination and defecation.

Autonepiophilia This term, from the Greek "autos" (self) "nepon" (infant) and "philia" (attachment), was coined by sexologist Professor John Money.[4] It refers to diaper fetishism in connection with transvestism and masochism as distinct from paraphilic infantilism.

I should also disambiguate two Freudian terms that sometimes crop up in age play circles that may appear to be more relevant than they actually are: anaclitism and psychosexual infantilism.

Anaclitism The ancient Greek word "ἀνακλίνω" or "anaklino", meaning "to lean against, to lean upon" was adopted by German, Freudian psychoanalysts and adapted into the word "Anlehnung", which was then translated into the English "anaclisis". The term refers to the act of obtaining sexual arousal from the objects and behaviors that one was exposed to as an infant. This doesn't mean age play activities. It means that sexual instincts developed out of self-preservation instincts. For example, Freudian psychology postulates that "[t]he infant's bodily function of simple hunger, to take a primary example, is at first attached solely to the act of suckling at mother's breast."[5] This act of nursing would, in keeping with this theory, later develop into a sexual proclivity to suck at a partner's nipple. Despite numerous misunderstandings of this outdated theory, it does not mean to eroticize being treated like a baby or nursery objects.

Psychosexual infantilism Dr. Sigmund Freud introduced this term to describe a condition in which individuals had not taken the usual route through psychosexual development to heterosexual maturity. It is sometimes confused with paraphilic infantilism, partly because of the similarities between the terms and partly because in his book, *Patterns of Psychosexual Infantilism*,[6] Dr. Wilhelm Stekel focused on cases that involved age play and diapers. Perhaps this exhibited his own misunderstandings of the paraphilia or perhaps it was a convenient metaphor for what was considered the immature development of a person's sexuality.

The point of medical texts is often to pathologize the people who are their subjects, which is why certain other medical terms, like those for a crossdresser or a transwoman which I will not repeat here, have come to be seen as offensive. Medical and psychological definitions are also based on individuals whose interests are developed to the point of obsession or who are ashamed of and feel the need to eradicate their fetishes and other aspects of their personalities. Keep these points in mind when resorting to psychological or medical texts to define yourself or your interests. Certain material might be useful to you, but proceed with caution!

I think that one of the reasons people remain interested in medical definitions despite their limitations is that many of us want to know where our desire to age play comes from or, in medical jargon, the etiology. As of yet, there's no definitive answer to this question, either accepted by the medical community or by the age play community itself.

Still, if we can't really answer the question, *Why do I age play?*, we can certainly answer the question, *What's enjoyable about age playing?* Below are some varied and relatable examples of what someone might like about engaging in age play.

- Enjoying a unique version of filial love for a partner in a caretaker role.
- Experiencing an altered, more childlike and wondrous state of consciousness.
- Feeling as though you're being your true self.
- Feeling cute.
- Feeling protected by one's caretaker.
- Feeling secure in a juvenile or familial setting.

- Not having to say goodbye to an enjoyable phase of your life.
- Relief from responsibility.
- Relief from worry.
- Reliving traumatic events in a positive way. (Note that if therapeutic age play has the power to heal, it also has the power to hurt, so be careful.)
- Stress reduction.

These are terms that can have a highly personal meaning and while it's extremely important to share common definitions of them and understand what a person in general might enjoy about age playing so as to begin to relate to a group's humanity, most of us are mainly interested in relating to each other on a personal level, and finding people who can know and understand us as we really are, perhaps because they are the same. So, now that we're all more or less on the same page (I hope), we can start to talk about defining age play in an immediately personal way: we can take a crack at defining our Little selves.

Defining Your Little Self

Some age players have a single, strongly-developed Little persona. Others have multiple personae in various stages of development.

Some of us view our age play persona as a variable expression of ourselves, which may not require much or even any development. Even if you don't feel the need to develop or define your own Little persona, you may want to understand how others go about it. Perhaps it will help you to better introduce playmates to your Little side.

There are an infinite number of ways to define your age play persona because the nuances of personality are infinite. It's an extremely personal undertaking, and definitions intended for across-the-board application can be so open-ended as to be meaningless. That said, many people do benefit from some sort of definition. If nothing else, it helps us to begin to communicate with each other.

You may not like labels, but you're going to have a hard time expressing yourself without some sort of shared vocabulary. Language is a tool. Instead of letting it limit you, use it to your advantage, if only to build a jumping off point for conversations with potential playmates.

Not everyone is opposed to labels, though. Some people seem to always be searching for that flawless micro-label that is all-encompassing, perfectly personalized, and exclusive of everything that they are not. These words don't always exist for everyone, at least not in modern English, or they may only apply to a small part of someone's personality. I'm more than just an age play switch. Even when I tell someone that I'm a cisgender, femme Mommy-babygirl brat switch who bottoms to my Daddy Dom and tops my collared, submissive Little boy, they're not going to automatically get a completely accurate idea of my sexual psyche and what my relationships look like, but it is a starting place. We're still going to need to have a conversation, probably quite a few, to make sure that we're more or less understanding each other.

On that note, I find that sit-down-and-get-to-know-you conversations aren't always the best way to sit down and get to know someone. Unplanned, natural, recurring conversations over a long period of time are often more revelatory and allow for a more genuine connection. Of course, they require a much larger investment of time.

The desire to add legitimacy to your Little persona by claiming to be a "true" age player, Little, babygirl, etc. doesn't help anyone. To be blunt, it's putting on airs. People can change drastically or not when they are being Little. If someone doesn't age play in the way that you do and that's a problem for you, don't question the validity of their identity: just leave them alone and do your own thing.

Maybe it makes sense that we Littles and kinksters are so picky about our labels. We're supposed to be able to define ourselves as clearly as any other subculture. Atheists don't believe in the super-natural. Mycologists are interested in fungi. Francophiles like French stuff. There's a lot more at stake for age players (and other kinksters), too. After all, people don't go around making assumptions about how good or bad a mycologist's childhood was based solely on their interest in mushrooms. We've got a lot riding on this label. It would be nice if we could get it just right in an easy, one-word, universally-understood answer, but some in-depth explanation is usually necessary.

As you encounter various age play, sexual, romantic, and kink identities, remember that even terms and labels that seem gendered are not inherently so. Just as you define your own gender, you ultimately determine all of which personal identity labels apply to you. A Daddy Dom is nothing more than someone who likes to be called a Daddy Dom. A babygirl is nothing more than someone who likes to be called a babygirl. Perhaps you enjoy a label specifically *be-cause* it clashes with your gender identity or presentation. During sex, I really enjoy calling femme tops "Daddy"--assuming that they let me. It feels subversive and gives them a good idea of what sort of play I like.

People are mostly curious and may ask questions if your label does-n't seem like it fits in with what they have assumed about you. These people are sometimes (even oftentimes) being rude and argumentative upon encountering something that they don't understand. Other times people are just trying to get to know you and would really appreciate your efforts, should you feel like making them.

If you get asked over and over again about your identity, instead of changing it to suit others, you might want to have a standard response ready so that you can answer basic questions. Alternatively, you can be more selective about with whom you discuss your identity, only opening up to a few people who are likely to understand you better without as much of an explanation. Then again, you may *enjoy* talking about yourself! Remember that others have these feelings, too, and be respectful of their personal decisions.

Few people remain unchanged their whole lives. Don't be afraid to embrace your changing identity. It doesn't invalidate earlier incarnations of your personality. Phases of consciousness and identity are, in my opinion, one of the great joys in life. Do you--all of you. If, conversely, you take joy in a single, life-long identity, good for you! Stasis and fluidity are both beautiful in their own ways. Just don't be a jerk about it.

You can certainly mention how you may not fit perfectly under a certain label, but don't forget to mention how that label *does* work for you, or the rest of us will wonder why you're using it. Don't assume that we'll know! It also makes you seem more positive and approachable. You could only say, "I'm a Little, but I don't like coloring or cuddling." It's much more helpful if you follow it up with, "And I'm really into cartoons, gothic lolita clothes, and being spanked when I'm naughty!" It lets potential friends and play partners know what we might do to engage you and allows us to see positive similarities in our identities.

If you feel that you need some help starting those conversations, below are some questions to ask yourself that might help you to explain the who, what, when, where, and why of your Little persona to others. You could even use these questions as writing prompts for journal entries or an essay. Posting publicly on a blog or vlog will also help you to get out there and meet other people who share your interest in age play. In addition, such musings can make a handy tool for negotiating with playmates or just help you to feel your Little self more strongly.

You can answer these questions more than once, perhaps for each Little persona that you have or for each age that you like to roleplay. Feel free to answer questions by explaining how they don't apply to you and to add your own, more relevant questions to the list. Think about what your audience (yourself, an ideal partner, your current partner, the age play community, etc.) should know about your Little self and remember that you don't have to discuss everything all at once. Think about what you might like to know about the person you're talking to and remember that they may not be ready to disclose everything, even if you are.

Last, but not least, remember that answers may change over time or differ depending on with whom you're interacting. Don't be afraid to contradict yourself later. It can be frustrating for your partner, but communication should always be ongoing. A good partner will never use what you said before to pressure you to do something that you've recently decided that you don't like, or to make you adhere to an identity that no longer works for you.

Who is your Little self?

Behavior

- When in Little mode, do you behave yourself?
- Which adjectives describe you? Are you bratty? Helpful? Shy?
- Does your behavior and demeanor heavily depend on the situation?

Label

- Are there any labels that might help others to understand you better?
- Do you like this label?
- What, if anything, do you wish was different about how

people perceived the label?

- Do you use this label only out of necessity or do you wear it proudly?

Personality

- Do you have a Little personality distinct from your everyday self? If so, what are the differences?
- Do you prefer being your everyday self to being Little or vice versa? Do you enjoy both personas more or less equally?

Regression

- Do you like to regress, i.e. feel like you've become a younger age, when you're age playing? If so, how do your behavior and thoughts change?
- If you do regress, is your Little self an expression of an alternate personality, or just you as your younger self?

What does your Little like to do?

Clothing

- What sort of clothing does your Little like to wear? Do you like special panties, ruffled socks, onesies, overalls, etc.?
- Do you consider age play clothes to be fetish wear or would you wear them in public in your daily life?

- Would you be able to age play without these clothes?

Companionship

- Do you enjoy playing with other Littles?
- Are your relationships with other Littles an expression of polyamory or are they strictly platonic?
- Do you enjoy being cared for by caregivers who may not be bonded to you, like a babysitter, or do you only want a very close caregiver, like a Mommy?
- List three characteristics of the ideal Big for your Little.
- List three characteristics of your Little's perfect best friend.

Diapers

- Do you like to wear diapers when you're being Little? If so, what kind? (Birdseye cloth diapers, disposable diapers, training pants, etc.)
- Are you loyal to a particular brand?
- Choose three adjectives to describe your perfect diaper.
- Do you like to use diapering toiletries like baby powder, baby oil, petroleum jelly, diaper rash cream, etc.?
- Do you become embarrassed when you wear a diaper and, if so, is it enjoyable to be embarrassed?
- Do you like wetting or messing your diaper? If so, do you like being made to wear a wet or soiled diaper for an exten-

ded length of time?

- What are the steps of your ideal changing ritual?
- Is a diaper change sexual for you? If so, is it foreplay or the main event? Is a diaper itself a sex toy to you?
- How do you feel about simulated messy diapers with things like shaving cream or bananas?
- Do you enjoy forced diaper use, like enemas and diuretics? Be specific.
- How do you feel about including sexual paraphernalia like butt plugs in a diaper change?

Play

- What are your Little self's favorite things to do during play-time?
- Do you have any special toys? Would you be upset if someone else touched or used this toy?
- Are you good at sharing?
- Would you engage in an activity that you didn't like or found boring in order to accommodate a playmate?
- Describe a perfect afternoon with your ideal Little best friend.
- Do you have imaginary friends? Are you friends with your stuffed animals and toys?

Punishment

- Does your Little self enjoy or tolerate being punished?
- Would you prefer punishments to be humiliating, painful, or time-consuming?
- Which punishments would you absolutely not submit to?
- How does being punished make you feel?
- Should punishment be an experience on its own or only in response to misbehavior on your part?
- Would you become upset or defiant if you felt that you were being punished unjustly?
- List five punishments that you would enjoy submitting to.
- Should punishments be appropriate to your Little age? What are your criteria for determining appropriate punishment?

Rules

- Do you enjoy having special rules for when you're in Little space?
- Are these rules meant to control your behavior or help you get into Little space?
- Would these rules be realistic rules that a chronological child should abide by, like washing your hands before you eat, or fetishistic, like having to wet at least two diapers per day?
- Would these rules be set by your Big alone or would you have input? Are there certain rules that you would not con-

sent to?

- Based on your Little age, how much control would a Big have over you in regards to leisure time, goals, speech, dress, hygiene, etc.? For example, someone playing as one-year-old probably would not dress themselves, but a twelve-year-old may exclusively make decisions about their dress.

Work

- Does your Little self have chores? Homework? If so, do you have a good attitude about it?
- Do you enjoy using age play in order to motivate you to do work, like having a sticker chart or earning a reward?
- Would this scenario work only in a fantasy setting or would you like to be motivated to complete mundane chores, like paying bills and cleaning the kitchen?

When and where do you like to be Little?

Frequency

- How often do you like to age play?
- Do you always like to go "all the way" or is it sometimes preferable to experience a lighter, less immersive age play, like only sucking on a pacifier or just wearing age play clothes?
- Are there certain things going on in your life that might make

you want to age play more or less often or is your desire pretty constant?

Location

- Are there certain places that make you feel more Little?
- Are there spaces that you feel are sacrosanct only to age play or only to being Big? If so, why?
- Are there any changes that can be made to a space to make it feel more like a safe or fun place for you to be Little, like making sure the space is soundproof or putting out nursery décor?

Public

- Are you comfortable age playing in vanilla, non-adult settings, like the zoo?
- Do you like to age play in semi-public settings, like at a BDSM play party?
- If you do play in public, what's your plan for dealing with onlookers who may become curious, uncomfortable, or offended?

Impetuses

- Is there something that can happen that makes you feel Little?

- Do you enjoy it when something unexpectedly makes you feel Little? Can it be deliberately initiated?
- Is it embarrassing to be made to feel Little in public, even if you aren't acting Little?

Why do you like to be Little?

Dominance

- Is your Little side always or sometimes dominant?
- Do you feel dominant toward everyone or only to a specific person or type of person?
- Is your Little mean, like a bully or a tattletale?
- Is your Little a leader?

Masochism

- Do you enjoy physical discomfort when in Little space, like spankings, hair-pulling, rough penetration, etc.?
- Do you enjoy emotional discomfort, like being teased, being scolded, being put on time out, losing your favorite toy, etc.? If so, is this discomfort just part of your interactions as a Little or is it a punishment?
- Should punishments be non-sexual, sexual, or a mix of the two?
- Do you enjoy more domestic punishments like being

spanked with a belt or hairbrush?

- Do you enjoy more institutional punishments like being spanked with a paddle or being made to hold dictionaries on outstretched arms?

Romance

- Does your Little self experience full-blown feelings of adult love or crushes?
- How would your Little self express romantic affection?
- In which ways would you not like to experience or express romantic affection as a Little? Would these expressions make you uncomfortable or do they just not resonate with you?
- Is your Little self more or less open to multiple romantic re-lationships than your Big self? Equally open?
- Is it appropriate for a Little your age to have a romantic part-ner and go on dates? Would you do it even if or because it was inappropriate?
- Would your partner take the lead in the relationship or would you?
- Would you only date your Big?
- Would your relationship to your Big be more of a parent-child relationship where your Big would determine whether or not you could date other individuals?

Sadism

- Does your Little self like to hurt others? If so, why? (If your Little side is indeed sadistic, you may want to visit Wikipedia's entry, *List of School Pranks*.[7])
- Do you enjoy inflicting physical pain, like giving someone a wedgie or an Indian burn?
- Do you enjoy inflicting emotional pain, like calling someone names or insisting that a Big read you a sexual story when they don't want to?

Sex

- Do you like to have sexual contact when in Little space? If so, what kind? Do you like to masturbate in Little mode?
- Does play still feel sexual even if you're not engaging in sexual activity?
- Do you like the vibe to feel intense, playful, coerced, or some other way?
- Do you prefer to be the one to initiate sexual contact? How might your partner ask if you would like to be sexual and obtain consent?
- What, if anything, makes a sexual experience as a Little different from a sexual experience as a Big?

Stress

- Does entering Little headspace allow you to de-stress or experience emotions that you might usually have trouble accessing?
- Are there things that can stress you out when you're Little?
- How does your Little respond to stress?

Submission
- As a Little, do you feel submissive to certain people, for example, caregivers?
- Do you only feel submissive to one person? Are you submissive in general?
- Is being made to be Little the same as being made to submit?

What age do you like to play?

You may have noticed that I haven't mentioned age very often in my questions about how you like to age play. I'm going to include some questions about your age play age just in case you might want them, but I want to more deeply discuss how age figures into age play, because I think that this fundamental connection has been poorly developed.

Most people will first mention their Little side's age and gender when attempting to define their age play personas. Just as gender is often best expressed on a spectrum, I believe that each specific age is also best expressed on a spectrum.

Age play age is actually more difficult to nail down than most people assume. For one thing, a lot of age players don't have extensive (or any) experience with chronological children of the age that they like to roleplay and even fewer are child development specialists.

For argument's sake, let's say that someone *is* a child development specialist well-versed in the developmental stage that they are age playing. Does remembering to, say, suppress the pincer grasp, but still use the palmar grasp in order to present being a five-month-old help them get lost in the roleplay or is it just distracting and unnatural? Not to mention things that you can't emulate, like having as many neural synapses as a two-year-old. It's just impossible.

Specific roleplay age may not be a very useful means of definition anyway. One person's "nine" is very different from another's. Are all thirty-year-olds developmentally alike? Not remotely. At thirty, I have two kids, a partner, an ex-husband, my own business, and two books out. At thirty, my Little boy Sam Solo has been to numerous foreign countries, had tons of life experiences that I can only dream of, has no children, and has never been married. Different people linger on or skip different milestones.

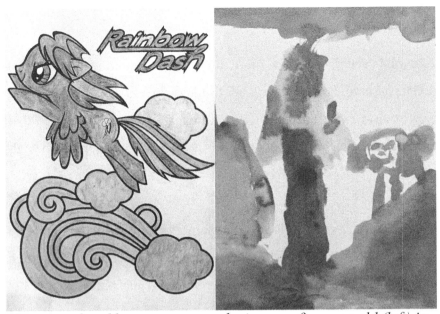

Picture colored by a person age playing as a five-year-old (left) in comparison to a picture painted by a chronological five-year-old (right) because I couldn't convince them to use a coloring book.

Age ranges, like "teenager" or "toddler", may be more useful. Even within those parameters, I often see people borrowing from ages very different from their own, like an age player who likes to be seven contently and unquestionably using a baby bottle. I would expect an actual child of that age to have been using a cup for quite some time--assuming that there were no developmental issues that made it impractical to do so. But, hey! It's a roleplay! Have fun with it!

Even better than giving your range is a well-thought-out and clear description of *why* you want to portray a certain age. Did you really, really like being six-years-old? Are you very interested in experiencing the types of limitations that you feel are appropriate for a child of twelve?

Age range

- Which age ranges do you like to roleplay?
- Are these age ranges expressions of the same persona or is, say, your teenager persona completely separate from your toddler persona?

Perception of the age

- List ten adjectives that you feel strongly represent this age. They may also apply to other ages. (Examples: innocent, sweet, playful, shy, inquisitive, dependent, vulnerable, bossy, curious, sassy.)
- Is there a fictional character who you feel represents this age really well?

Personal history (Note that some people are not comfortable discussing this at all. You may want to skip these questions entirely if they bother you.)

- When you were this age, what was your life like?
- What were you like?
- How do you wish these things were different? What did you enjoy?

- What do you feel it is important for Bigs to know about Littles playing this age?

Labels

Below are some labels common in the age play world and what most people will mean when they use them. People often argue over terms and definitions, but you can turn an argument into a discussion and even learn from it! Even if these were words that had been formalized in the Oxford dictionary, definitions are still full of nuances, as well as subject to regional and other inconsistencies.

Adult baby/little boy/little girl/kid/toddler Someone who role-plays or regresses to a younger age, usually reflective of the age mentioned in the label. Note that *adult baby*, *adult little boy*, *adult little girl*, and *adult kid* are sometimes abbreviated to AB, ALB, ALG, and AK, respectively.

Babyfur or cub As it sounds, a babyfur or cub is a furry version of an age player, usually diapered. A furry is a person who enjoys wearing full, mascot-style fursuits, or perhaps just furry heads, hands, and feet or any combination of those accessories. If you're having trouble picturing a furry, imagine a cute, cartoon-style, anthropomorphic animal--real or fantastical--rendered in a costume. There are variations, but that image should get you most of the way until you can manage to look it up online.

Babygirl or babyboy Though "baby" is in the label, babygirls and babyboys are sometimes more toddler-age or even teenage roleplayers. This may not be an age play term at all, but only refer to someone who is submissive, perhaps with a cute aesthetic.

Big Someone, perhaps a caregiver or authority figure, who interacts with age players by assuming an adult role. Sometimes, someone will refer to their Big personality in order to differentiate between their non-age play persona and their Little self. (You may need to clarify which definition you are invoking in conversation.)

Brat An age player who may be naughty, mean, or sassy on purpose, possibly to goad a Big or caregiver into punishing them, as a way of being dominant while still being Little, or perhaps in order to better top from the bottom.

Caregiver A Big who watches over and provides care and entertainment for age players.

DD/lg Abbreviation for "Daddy Dom/little girl"; a Dominant/submissive (D/s) relationship in which the Daddy is dominant over the submissive little girl, who may be more of a childlike adult than regressive roleplayer. Mommy Dom(me)/little boy, Daddy Dom/little boy, and Mommy Dom(me)/little girl are responsive terms, though they are not as widely used at this time.

Kidz Age players who roleplay as elementary- or high school-age children.

Kitten or pet Pet play can be very distinct from age play, but there are regressive, sometimes submissive players who prefer playing as some sort of cuddly creature. Kittens and other pets will often wear only ears, possibly with paws, tails, collars, or other smaller costume items while babyfurs and furries will don full fursuits or full-head masks. Furries may be interested in D/s as well, but the D/s dynamic is definitive of kittens and pets. If you are unsure whether a person is a furry or a pet, you can ask them, assuming that it is appropriate to do so--or just don't worry about it.

Little An age player who assumes the role of a child. Alternately, a childlike adult who chooses to identify themselves with this term.

Lolita Someone who identifies with the "nymphette" persona described by Nabokov in his book, *Lolita*. Lolitas are adults who usually roleplay as pre-teen to teenage children.

Middle An age player who plays a slightly older age, like a pre-teen or teenager.

Sissy A man who likes to be dressed up in hyperfeminine and perhaps hyper-childish attire as a form of power exchange or as part of humiliation play.

Accessing Little Space

Once you've defined your Little self, or at least started to, how can you consistently get into the right headspace? Naturally, it should be a lot easier once you know what it is, but it can still take some work. One of the reasons it's useful to have a good, strong definition of your Little self is so that you can gauge whether or not you've successfully gotten into that headspace and make adjustments for an even more immersive experience next time.

For a long time, I would go to events and realize that, while I had a good time, I may not have been in Little space--or perhaps the opposite was true. After all, sometimes I'm feeling sad or grumpy--and so is my Little self. The point is: am I feeling emotions *as my Little self?*

Stable headspace is good for you, your play partner, and those around you. I used to have a partner who was constantly in and out of headspace and, let me tell you, playing with her was not fulfilling. "I'm Big! I'm Little! I'm Big! Now I'm Little!" all within a few minutes. It was so dizzying that eventually I stopped caring which headspace she was in because I certainly wasn't experiencing the one that I wanted to be in.

It's especially considerate to do your best to maintain your headspace if you're age playing in a large group and helping to establish a mood at an event. And be mindful of helping your Big get into their headspace, just as they're mindful of helping you!

The three ways that I like to get myself and others into headspace are:

1. Bonded objects
2. Immersive roleplay
3. Hypnosis or guided meditation

Bonded object If you're a physical sort of person, taking a special object and using it only when you're age playing can help strengthen your sense of your Little self. You can start using a bonded object in one or both of two ways: using the object when you happen to feel Little or using the object during age play sessions. The first way is usually a lot harder, especially if your bonded object is something that you can't just have around all the time. It's unlikely that you can dash off to some private spot to slip into a diaper in the middle of work. It may also be awkward to explain why you have it, should it be discovered as you go about your daily routine.

I find that it's usually more practical for most people to set aside some time to do something regressive, like watching a cartoon or receiving a spanking, and then using the object. I admit that it's less organic, but since most of us aren't able to run around age playing at will, most age play is probably going to be planned anyway. Eventually doing age play activities in the company of this object will help you to start associating it with age play itself. You'll start to learn that having this object means that it's time to be Little.

Examples of potential bonded objects:
- Baby key chain toy, rattle, or other baby toy
- Bib
- Blankie
- Bottle or sippy cup
- Diapers
- Doll, teddy bear, or other stuffie
- Cute clothes, like hair bows, saddle shoes, onesies, etc.
- Pacifier or teether
- Panties or underwear in a juvenile style
- Plastic pants
- School uniform

While you may specifically want your bonded object to be age play-related, it doesn't have to be. A length of ribbon, a bell, a smooth stone--anything can work really. I often wear some rhinestone safety pin earrings when age playing, but at no other time. I've noticed that they've become a sort of unintentional age play impetus.

Immersive roleplay Immersive roleplay takes you completely out of your everyday world. People treat you differently and your surroundings have changed, making it difficult for you not to go along with the world you find yourself in. I use this technique most often in my professional sessions. After all, we're in a location used exclusively for this purpose, almost as though the entire house were one all-encompassing bonded object. We're both dressed differently than usual and using terms that we may never even say aloud except in each other's presence. And of course we both really want to lose ourselves in the experience!

I had one professional partner who was particularly concerned about his ability to get into a roleplay scene, even though he desperately wanted to. I told him that I was sure that it would be fine. He was to be playing my son and I was to be his mom. We met, had a brief in-person negotiation, and decided to dive right in. I began berating him for some transgression and, as he had suspected, he was having trouble getting into headspace. In fact, he was laughing in my face.

Instead of ending the scene and going back to negotiation or ignoring it and trying to push through, I did what I would have done if I really was a strict 1950s mom whose nine-year-old was laughing in my face while I was trying to scold him: I hauled him into the kitchen, pulled a fresh bar of ivory soap from my apron pocket, lathered it up, and proceeded to wash his mouth out. "Do you still think I'm funny?" His demeanor immediately changed and he was able to lose himself as never before.

I should note that while the mouth soaping was not specifically negotiated, we did talk about a safeword and I gave him ample time to use it as I took him into the kitchen, talked about what I was going to do, unwrapped the soap, and so on. In-scene negotiation is a wonderful skill for tops and bottoms alike to develop.

Hypnosis or guided meditation Bonded objects can also be used in connection with hypnosis and guided meditation. Whole books have been written on hypnosis and how to be a good subject. It's a very broad topic that can only be partially explored here, but even just lying in a calm, dim room and focusing on regression can help you to lose yourself in Little space.

If there is someone available who can talk you through a guided meditation or hypnosis session, great! If not, you can still do this on your own.

Either way, try to take the time to set up your room first. I like to use a baby powder scent to make the room seem more like a nursery. They say that scent is the sense most strongly tied to memory, and I like to think that the smell helps to remind me and my playmate of other times we've had a successful age play session. I also like to have the lights turned down, as most people have trouble focusing when there's a light glaring through their closed eyes. Being of a comfortable temperature and not being hungry or needing to use the restroom should help as well. All you're trying to do is minimize distractions, even though you probably can't eliminate them completely.

When you go into your session, remember to focus on the experience more than on your body. You're trying to get into Little space, not stay perfectly still. If you have an itch, scratch it. If you need to cough, cough. If you have your bonded object with you, feel free to suck on that pacifier or cuddle that teddy bear! Let your body take care of itself so that you can focus on your actual task.

If you have someone who can hypnotize you or talk you through your meditation, discuss what you're trying to accomplish with them thoroughly. They can describe an age play scenario for you or talk about how you want to feel as a Little. They can be suggestive or forceful, as you feel is best. Don't over-analyze what they say and know that you two can have a conversation after the session is over on ways to make next time even better.

If you don't have a partner or just want to do it yourself, you can imagine a guide who is doing those things for you, record yourself in advance, purchase a pre-made or custom recording, or just fantasize. Feel free to experiment with different techniques and try to find what works for you.

Maintaining Little headspace can be difficult for some age players. Specific triggers may jar you out of it or it might just dissipate. If something is happening to pull you back into adult headspace, you can either try to avoid the distraction or re-interpret it as something that makes you feel Little. Perhaps people asking you to make decisions pulls you out of headspace. Instead of going back into adult mode, you could practice responding as your Little self would, even if that means just shuffling your feet, staring at your toes, and mumbling, "I don't know."

If you're unsure of what is harshing your Little buzz, I would recommend engaging in shorter bursts of age play where you know that you'll be able to maintain headspace, with a set decision for what you'll do when Little time is over. Perhaps you just play with your toys for 10 minutes, then go back into adult mode by taking a shower. Add time to your age play sessions until they're as long as you would like them to be and always have an ending ritual to mark the difference between Little you and Big you.

While we're at it, let's discuss coming out of Little space. Some players are amazing at slipping into Little headspace, but not so amazing at coming back to the adult world. Decide how you would like to feel when coming out of Little space, whether you would like to just float back to adulthood or whether you would like a crisper ending. One of the ways to end your age play scene is with aftercare that focuses on adult behavior, like having a cocktail or reading an adult book.

community

History

The Littles community is growing every day. Many people cite the internet as the catalyst that set the community to booming. We seem to be experiencing a surge in the Littles population and while the internet is certainly an important tool for organizing, educating, and connecting, it didn't cause that surge. It's easy to give something so revolutionary as the internet credit for just about every modern phenomenon, but in my opinion the current age play surge is the result of a shift in our culture that prizes a childlike outlook on life. While most people settle for adult coloring books and bars with video games, a special few take a step further into actual age play.

As noted in Paul Rulof's *Ageplay: From Diapers to Diplomas*, "long before the Web, long before Windows, before Mac's [sic], before

DOS, almost before the first commercial personal computers were available, there was DPF."[1] DPF was originally known as Diaper Pail Fraternity, but as the gay men's group began attracting a wider variety of sexual orientations and genders, the name was changed to Diaper Pail Friends. DPF was started in 1980 by a man named Tommy as a mailing list and newsletter, but grew into a now inoperative age play supplies company and internet presence at dpf.com. DPF's move towards online communication began around 1991. You can view previous incarnations of the website as early as 1996 by entering the URL at archive.org/web.

Some sources claim that Tommy didn't recognize the value of a three-letter URL and just let it go in 2010 instead of either selling or developing it--assuming that he hasn't passed away. Other sources claim that the site went down in 2008 as Tommy's health declined and that he and his partner, Markie, were holding out for an unrealistically large sum.[2] (I was quoted $175,000 just for the URL.) Whatever happened, dpf.com now sits unused, forlorn, and expensive.

Other pre-internet abdl presences include Infantae Press's fetish magazines, including *The Play Pen*, *Tales from the Baby Room: Bizarre Stories for the Adult Baby*, and *Adults in Babyland*. Infantae was established by Cathy Slovik, born Charles. This Seattle-based transwoman also published items for crossdressers and transwomen under the Empathy Club.

Amber Enterprises, or Amber E. for short, was run by a woman named Florence, who passed away in 1997. Amber E. produced the first exclusively adult baby-themed magazine, *The Play Pen*, which was initially published around 1975 and subsequently taken over by Infantae in 1979. Amber E. began producing a newsletter titled *Crib Sheet* in 1976.[3] Amber E. would eventually transform into the now closed Very Special Clothes, run by Florence's niece, known as Auntie V.

Thumb was an adult baby magazine from the good people who published the mainstream adult magazine *Finger*. Adult babies and diaper lovers would also show up in alternative magazines such as the infamous *Fetish Times* and *Nugget* or write into advice columns like Xaviera Hollander's "Call Me Madam" in *Penthouse*. *Rubber Life* and *Rubber Nurse* magazines occasionally offered ABDL stories by Nurse Linda Latex.

Adult babies and diaper fetishists could also attempt to connect through professional sex workers who would occasionally host events or facilitate playdates. An episode of an old documentary-style show, *British Sex*, shows a group of older men engaging Nanny Dawson to attend their age play party.[4] Dated as it is, the party, given by a man named Richard, with its sissy maid, cocktails, adorable clothes, and spankings, looks like something that I would definitely enjoy!

The purchasing of age play clothing and accouterments presented another way for age players to connect pre-internet. Mommy Carolyn of Carolyn's Kids offered a mail order catalogue (which likely just as often served as makeshift pornography) as well as an in-person shopping experience in her Melrose, Massachusetts home. HB Enterprises, also known as Precious Babywear and established in 1986 by Mummy Hazel, was the English equivalent. NK Products, based out of New Jersey, offered a newsletter, *Adult Baby World*, in addition to age play clothing and adult diapers. The Little Rascals, an ABDL fetish clothing company in the United Kingdom, went a step further and hosted monthly club get-togethers.

But all this was clandestine, underground stuff. The public got a glimpse of ABDL play in the early 1990s when ABDLs started appearing on talk shows like *the Jerry Springer Show* and *the Montel Williams Show*. The response was what was to be expected, with callers and audience members condemning age players and diaper fetishists to hell and calling them pedophiles. Shows sometimes attempted to be more educational than sensational. San Francisco sexologist Dr. Charles Moser was invited to appear on *The Phil Donahue Show* to provide an unbiased, generally positive perspective-- but it wasn't enough.

The Phil Donahue Show also featured Gene Smith, who founded the Great Lakes Adult Diaper Society (GLADS), another pre-internet ABDL group. Other notable players of this era included Kent Perry and Christopher Taylor who organized ABDL parties all across America. Kent's short, but information-packed autobiography is available on understanding.infantilism.org.

Married couple Jean and Don Davis wrote and took pictures for Diaper Pail Friends until Jean was killed in a car accident in 1989. Angela Bauer, a semi-closeted lawyer with incontinence issues and an interest in spanking subsequently married Don and they became the new, straight ABDL power couple. Angela retained her maiden name to avoid confusion with another lawyer, Angela Davis. Angela would take over many of the roles previously filled by Jean, appearing on talk shows and in ABDL fetish videos. She is currently living in Pasadena.

Big Babies, Infantilists, and Friends (bbif.org), which is still around, was an early internet embodiment of the community which was founded in 1993. A Usenet newsgroup, alt.sex.fetish.diapers (ASFD), was the early go-to for chatting with other ABDLs. (Newsgroups were social media predecessors that existed on the pre-world wide web internet.)

Going further back, there is evidence for the swelling of a main-stream, non-sexual, young-at-heart culture in the late 1800s and early 1900s. The Victorian cult of the child and the Edwardian era's more specific cult of the little girl were developed in literature such as *Alice's Adventures in Wonderland*, *Peter Pan*, and *The Wonderful Wizard of Oz*. In her blog article "The Victorian cult of the child", Eni Elisa Hausmann wrote that, "Due to an utter dedication to child-hood...[the authors] seemed to unfold their engrained desire to be an innocent child."[5] Interestingly, *Alice's Adventures in Wonderland* was first published about the time the phrase "young at heart" came into use in the mid-19th century.

The characters from these stories have endured the years at least partly because of their depiction of adults in child form, empowered with physical independence, yet free of limiting responsibilities and preconceptions. Their minds are clear to experience and critique the world they encounter--to get into trouble and out of it again with a fluidity that many adults lack. We even see Wendy and Peter indulge a bit of D/s age play when they assume parental roles over the Lost Boys.[6] I like to think that these passages enable adult readers to simultaneously enjoy the normally incompatible pleasures of parent-hood and the simplicity of childhood.

Of course there have always been and always will be a few people interested in age play regardless of the current cultural state, but that number has definitely increased in recent years. Christopher Noxon's book *Rejuvenile: Kickball, Cupcakes, and the Reinvention of the American Grown-up*; Adrienne Raphel's New Yorker article "Why Adults are Buying Coloring Books (for Themselves)"; and Joseph Epstein's essay "The Perpetual Adolescent" all discuss these trends in how we adults perceive ourselves as well as our telling real-world actions.

I mention all these things to illustrate that the age play community, no matter what you call it, big or small, brazen or incognito, has existed for a long time. We found ways to connect before the internet, no matter how difficult that was. I only hope that someday someone is poring over outdated articles about the fetish and community and comes across my name!

Making Connections

The time is right for developing the Littles community. We have the will, we have the technology, and we have thousands of other people to do it with us. Once you've found your local community, you can begin the process of becoming part of it and adding to it. I'm going to give as much quantifiable advice as I can on how to do that, not because I want to raise up a legion of Little pick up artists, but because some of us need specifics. "Be yourself!" is a great tip, but, "Develop two useful or interesting hobbies and be able to talk about them," is much more practical.

Even if you're exclusively interested in private, monogamous play or only in borderline anonymous, no-strings-attached (NSA) play, I strongly recommend finding community instead of trying to find a single partner. Finding a stranger who is interested in exploring any type of relationship with you based heavily on shared sexual interests (and maybe some unflattering pictures of either your cock or a blurry closeup of your lips) is extremely difficult. In fact, you're probably ruining your chances with most people if that's all they can see of you, especially when someone else is doing things right and making you look bad by comparison.

Most people want to be valued as a whole person, even if they're just looking for play or a fling. You'll be more successful in the long term if you find a group of people who share your interest in age play, diapers, etc. and then...forget about all that! Focus instead on developing friendships--nothing more--with your fellow roleplayers and fetishists. Don't try to order up a play partner as you might order up a pizza unless you're willing to hire a professional. (And, hey, hiring a pro can be a lot of fun!)

If you are specifically participating in the community in order to find a playmate, you have to start knowing what it is that you're looking for. Do some soul searching about your ideal playmate.

Think about what you can offer them in return for what they offer you. One-sided relationships are rarely happy.

What kind of partner are you looking for? A Big, a Middle, or another Little? Are they a certain sexual orientation or gender? Perhaps they're asexual or genderless? Are their political or religious beliefs important to you? What types of activities do you imagine doing together? What adjectives would you use to describe your ideal partner? What adjectives do you use to describe yourself? Don't just think in positives here. No one is flawless and this isn't about being perfect; it's about being compatible.

You should also know if you're looking for a top or a dominant. A top is someone who takes control of their bottom partner in sexual situations. A dominant is someone who sets rules and protocol for their submissive's life. Or at least that's what those terms mean now, in most circles. Older players generally consider "top" to be an umbrella term for other players who take the guiding hand in the bedroom and "dominant" to mean a type of top who enjoys BDSM. So, do use these words if you feel that they're relevant, but make sure that you and your conversational companion are using the same meaning.

You may want to write a letter to an imaginary, ideal playmate. In it, you can tell them what you can do for them, why you feel that you two are a good match, and what you're excited about experiencing with them. If you find someone who makes you feel the same way that you felt writing that letter, you may have found a good match!

When you find someone who appears to fit the bill, be open and honest about your desires and expectations. That doesn't mean that you need to spill your guts on the first email exchange or even the first proper date. For example, just because you're looking for a long term relationship doesn't mean that you're not open to casually dating in the meantime. It's okay to just have fun and see what, if anything, develops.

When you're getting to know your potential playmate, you may want to ask them some questions. (And you should be able to answer these questions, too.)

- Have you been in an age play relationship before?
- What about your past relationships has been fulfilling?
- What about your past relationships has been difficult?
- What are you hoping to experience now?
- What are three accomplishments that you're proud of?
- What would you like to change about yourself and how do you plan to enact those changes?
- Could you share one of your recurring fantasies with me?
- What moved you to talk with me?

- How have you handled past breakups?
- Why do you want to get to know me?

Do you feel like they're just telling you what you want to hear? If you feel that they're manipulating you, you can just bow out of the conversation. If someone becomes abusive or threatening, don't hesitate to block them or even report them.

The point of asking these questions is to get to know the other person, not to get them to try on your Ideal Playmate Suit and see where you need to make alterations. You can have a fun and fulfilling relationship with someone who isn't perfect, but is largely compatible.

Online

It's hard to judge chemistry based only on emails and social media profiles, but that isn't to say that you need to take down your fetlife.com profile and only go to play parties. You can find community and relationships online, but instead of looking to meet a partner right off the bat, you'll have better luck establishing yourself through insightful forum posts; good, friendly pictures; and honest, well-written blog entries.

Why? Because people are savvy. They like to know what they're getting. That's why someone with numerous, diverse Instagram pics who participates in forum discussions gets tons of private messages while someone with no profile picture and a minimal About Me section will be left to wither. Your profile is a door-opener, like a resume. It helps people who don't know you at all get that all-important first impression of you.

Work on your community presence to make yourself desirable instead of essentially cold calling a bunch of people. You'll be starting real conversations, meeting active people, and making friends. There are huge online communities: forums, blogs, virtual worlds, and more. It's a jungle out there, which is really cool, but also why you should tread with care.

Take precautions online, especially if you're closeted. Remember that once a photo or video or other information snippet is out there, it's *out there*. Don't send pictures that you don't want to be seen. Remember that it's easy to lie and oftentimes the people who make you feel the most secure do so not because they're trustworthy, but because they know exactly how to appear to be trustworthy. If you can trust someone, you can trust them to not pester you for pictures or video of your face before you're ready to give them. Be careful on webcam shows, too, as they can be screenshot and even recorded.

You should already know this, too, but keep private information private. There's no good reason for someone to know your full legal name if you're only interacting online. As an adult actress, I know what it's like to have people pressuring you into giving your legal name, thinking that it will increase intimacy or put you into a vulnerable position. Don't fall for it. If you do want to share some information, invent a plausible pseudonym.

No matter where you go to find your online community, you're all but guaranteed to eventually be directed to fetlife.com. Even if you have no interest in BDSM, even if your Little is made of sunshine and lollipops and knows naught of darkness, you'll find yourself being directed to FetLife over and over again because it really is a well-designed, practical, collective resource. It's basically kinky Facebook.

Many online virtual world communities, like secondlife.com (SL), have drawn a number of age players because users (or "Residents") can employ a child avatar for a more immersive experience. If this sounds like something you would enjoy and are a sexual age player, know that SL prohibits "child avatars" from being in sexual situations. The SL wiki states that even "sexual content (sexual poseballs or equipment) in proximity to items traditionally associated with children (swing sets, etc.)" is forbidden.[7]

This is to protect them from being indicted under the PROTECT

Act, which prohibits computer-generated child pornography when "such visual depiction is a computer image or computer-generated image that is, or appears virtually indistinguishable from that of a minor engaging in sexually explicit conduct" (as amended by 1466A for Section 2256(8)(B) of title 18, United States Code). The Act doesn't say that it only applies to depictions of actual children, so it can be applied to illustrations of fictional children, drawings and sculptures--and pictures of drawings and sculptures.[8] No, you cannot say that, "It's supposed to be me, so it's okay!" I mean, you *can* say it, but it won't help you in court. The Act enables a maximum sentence of five years for possession and ten years for distribution of child pornography.

If you feel that you've wandered into a community that allows child pornography, even in the form of drawings or CGI, get out immediately and don't look back. There are plenty of online communities that don't include child porn. Also beware of people who simply claim a minor's age without clear and repetitive clarification that they are, indeed, adults. They may think that they're just age playing, but by not explicitly stating that they are only giving their role-play age, they may be unwittingly creating child porn. The laws are hazy, which is why you have to be extra careful!

Dating & No Strings Attached (NSA) Relationships

Are you specifically using social media to find a casual (NSA) play-mate or relationship? Have a plan: don't coerce or be overly aggressive. Your plan should allow you to measure your success and enjoyment, and hold you accountable to yourself for getting out there and making a real effort. Finding a playmate is fun, but it's also a task and the commodity you're looking for, whether a life-long partner or a one night stand, is rare and elusive.

First of all, I would suggest setting up a profile on at least three social media sites. I recommend fetlife.com, twitter.com, and tumblr.com. Forums and other sites that are more specialized to your interests, such as ddlgforum.com, are also a good idea. Engaging in multiple online communities not only spreads out your efforts, it helps to establish you as a recognizable figure. Also, you'll have something to link to in the links section. (Linking to other people's work makes you look like you have no accomplishments or anything worth sharing of your own. Just a tip.)

Take time writing your profile and run spellcheck. Proof read. I don't suggest overusing baby speak because it's easier to write than it is to read. You want your writing to be enjoyable, not another hurdle. That said, most people don't really read profiles, so keep it short and write lengthy blog entries instead.

Have some pictures on hand. Your initial profile picture should probably not be of your genitals, your diapered butt, your eyes, or your mouth--with or without a thumb or a pacifier. These pictures are generic and do not express anything individual or make an impression. You need to be unique if you want to be treated like you're unique. No one is impressed by diapered crotch pic number 6,147,865. Whenever I see an Instagram account that's nothing but a guy's diapered crotch or a woman's mouth with a pacifier in it, all I can think is, "Why bother having an account at all? The world has seen your one trick and it's boring."

I would also suggest staying away from cartoon characters or other pictures that aren't of you--unless you're a babyfur and it's art of yourself that you've commissioned or created. Instead of a picture of your favorite cartoon character or a pacifier as your profile picture, maybe a picture of you holding a stuffed animal version of that character or with the pacifier clipped to your cute outfit would be more humanizing. Remember: with social media you're trying to establish a connection over a machine, so humanize yourself as much as possible.

If you do want to use a picture that someone else created, ask their permission before posting it. Just offering to take it down if you get caught is not cool. Most people might not care, but it will make artists hate you. People will usually give their permission if asked, especially if you credit the image with a link. However, if someone doesn't give their permission, you're not entitled to use the image anyway. Take it gracefully and move on.

If you're comfortable showing your face, there are a number of articles written about profile pictures that different demographics tend to find titillating. A search engine or a trip to blog.okcupid.com can help you if you really want to go in depth, but basically, if you want to play the percentages, men are more attracted to pictures taken from a high angle that frame the chest, show the eyes looking at the camera, and depict the person smiling. In other words, dudes like the "MySpace pic." Lauren Urasek, the most messaged woman on OkCupid in New York, suggests taking pictures above eye-level, but only barely, which is also the ideal level for lighting. [9]

Women tend to be more attracted to pictures of people with neutral facial expressions who are not looking directly at the camera. [10] When making a neutral expression, I suggest trying to look like you're concentrating on something or relaxing. Try not to look angry or bored--and realize that this may take a couple of shots before you find yourself on the correct side of those fine lines.

Of course, articles analyzing these preferences tend to be cis- and heteronormative, meaning that they don't analyze the preferences of transgender, gay, non-binary, or queer people. Also, what is statistically the most popular may not correlate with what that one special person finds attractive. I quite enjoy pictures of both men and women smiling at the camera. I think it's cute.

If you want to place a personal ad, be sure to make it a good one. Most personal ads consist of someone's age and location and a few sexual demands. Your personal ad is not so much a place to list your sexual desires as where you can say what you can offer a partner or playmate.

Don't make it too long! A paragraph should be sufficient. Your personal ad is a way for people to get a sort of snapshot of you and decide if they want to go visit your profile to learn about you. Focus on describing what you offer, not what you want. Your tone should be fun, approachable, and conversational with an intriguing headline. You can mention your sexuality, but talk *about* it, don't just list fetishes or desires. "I'm into spanking, incest roleplay, and diapers," is a terrible ad. Instead try something like:

I enjoy the power dynamic inherent to Mommy-son roleplay, especially when paired with domestic discipline like mouth-soaping, spanking, caning, and erotic embarrassment. These other interests ultimately grow from my diaper fetish. I enjoy wearing and wetting disposable diapers on a more or less weekly basis, even as a top, and keep a good stock of Tykable diapers. I would be a good match for someone who enjoys diapering rituals with lots of baby powder and diaper rash cream. I like to feel a deep connection to the person that I'm changing, or to the person who is changing me. My bedroom is a full nursery, decorated with my favorite cartoon character, Winnie the Pooh. I like to baby talk to my playmate and tend to chatter a bit. I'm excited to develop a long-term relationship with a compatible person local to the San Francisco Bay Area.

Doesn't that give a much better idea of who the writer is? Doesn't it draw you in more? Just imagine if it was written for a real person!

Most people place personal ads to try to find a playmate more quickly, but they rarely lead anywhere. Personal ads are socially lazy and so the people who respond to them tend to be socially lazy, too, or giving into an impulse that they won't follow through on later when they're no longer aroused. A precious few are genuinely interested and interesting. But since it isn't like you've got anything to lose, it may be worth a shot, especially if you're feeling lucky!

If you've decided to set up a fetlife.com profile, the next step is to join some relevant groups and start contributing! Check community forums and groups at least once a week, preferably daily, and make a point of contributing something useful, i.e. providing requested information. Posts like, "Wanna Skype in 10 minutes?" or "Why can't I find a mommy?" don't generally help anyone. Again, think about what you can add to the community rather than what you can take from it.

If you're able to go out, set a deadline by which you must attend an event. It's more important that you go *somewhere* than that the event be a perfect match for you. It will help you practice being social in what may be an unusual setting to you, let you see what others are wearing and doing, and get people in the community to start recognizing you. Even if you spend your first few outings just staring at your shoes, get out there!

If you see something in a forum that resonates with you, mention it in a public comment. If you find that you're doing this over and over--at least five times--with one person in particular, you might want to send them a private message, mentioning that you really enjoy their perspective. Don't pressure them by saying that you want to chat further. That's clear by the fact that you've sent a PM and begging for social interaction is a huge turnoff for most people. Just focus on making a connection and be open to the possibility that it might not take. Handle disappointment gracefully and you'll not only leave yourself open for future interactions, but get a reputation for being chill and polite. Remember that particularly attractive or well-known people get many messages like this every day.

Better than random "I like your style!" messages are those which are based on a legitimate need to share information on a personal level.

These types of messages usually grow up around a real-world event, which is why you should get out there. In fact, these messages are by far the best way to make a connection with someone, so get involved!

If you have a blog, make an effort to post at least once a week. If you miss a week, dear god, don't write one of those, "Sorry it's been awhile since I updated..." blogs. They make you look more flakey than if you just skip a few posts. Remember to spell-check your writing and try to be positive.

If you're having trouble thinking of topics for entries, the newsletter email from submissiveguide.com often includes a journaling prompt that can be easily modified to apply to an age player. Try to include pictures or video in your blog. Of course pictures of yourself, happy and indulging in age play are best, but pictures of your toys, your nursery set up, or where you've gone on your age play outing are better than nothing. Make a list of other age play blogs to read and comment on a few posts here and there when appropriate.

Real World Safety

Before you meet someone in person, be sure to take necessary safety precautions. Just like anything else in life, dates can go horribly wrong and fortune favors the prepared.

Tell someone else about the meeting and where you'll be. Make sure that there's an e-paper trail, and tell your new friend that you've done these things. I like to try to get a legal name and a face picture at the very least. If someone isn't ready to give me these things, I don't meet with them alone. Instead, I invite them to a munch, party, or other public or semi-public event.

I do not give out my legal name to professional clients, and don't feel the need to. The point of doing so is to allow people to have a starting point in looking for you and they would have an easy enough time finding me, as I am a public figure, albeit a minor one. Don't let anyone pressure you into giving out information that you feel unsafe in sharing--just because someone gave you their legal name doesn't mean that you have to reciprocate, especially if they have no good reason for asking. It also doesn't mean that they have to meet with you, but safety first! There's only one you and we want to keep you safe!

If you're a 100-pound 18-year-old meeting with a 240-pound grown man, chances are he doesn't need to be worried about you knocking him out and dragging him to your car. This is about safety and fairness, not equality, and my best-guess, not-at-all-guaranteed advice on what is safest for you will vary according to your situation. Hence, if you are a large man looking to meet someone who may not be as physically powerful as you are, my advice would be to be more forthcoming with information, while still protecting yourself. A picture of your face can be given without giving someone the ability to blackmail you. Proof that you exist needn't equal proof that you are into age play.

Have a safety call--preferably not a text--set up afterwards with a code so that your contact will know whether or not you're in trouble. For example, if they ask you, "What do you want to do for dinner tonight?" and you say, "Definitely pizza," they'll know that you need them to call the cops immediately. Consider installing something like, "Find my iPhone" to track your phone and quickly alert friends, family, and authorities as to where you are--or at least where your phone is. You can also visit cuff.io for smart jewelry designed to notify your friends and family in the case of an emergency.

As for the actual meeting, have a clear agenda set. Are you meeting in Little mode? Are you just going to have coffee as adults? Are you going to meet ready to play just in case, but really just to talk things out? I always like to meet new people knowing that there's a possibility that we might play, but making it clear that we both have to agree to do so before we actually get into it.

Don't use pet names with the person you're meeting without their permission. Until you negotiate a power dynamic, they are not your "babyboy" or "Mommy." They are your equal.

You can end or avoid play while leaving things open for future inter-action. Be open to the other person taking the same route. Maybe things are just a little overwhelming this first time, but you would be open to the possibility of playing in a week or so. Maybe you're just not in the right headspace. Maybe you would like to tweak things over email before getting into it. Or maybe you have a policy of not playing on the first date. No matter your reason, you can like someone and still decide to take things slow, and the other person should be socially skilled enough to realize this.

As for where to meet, there are always the traditional locales: bars, coffee shops, restaurants. Here in San Francisco, we're lucky enough to have a kinky coffee shop, Wicked Grounds, that caters to age players. It's adults only and boasts a special Littles menu. A local park with a secluded spot where an intimate conversation might happen often sets the mood for age play while being relatively safe and creating no pressure. On a rainy day, a museum makes a worthy substitute. Again, you can always invite someone to a social event and meet among other people and lower the pressure even more.

If you and your potential play partner are active in the local community, you might want to ask around for references, either formally or casually. You don't have to be convinced that someone is a stalker rapist in order to be justified in vetting them. In fact, if you're convinced that they are, why would you bother? Asking around about someone's background and experience means that you're open to the idea that they might be totally cool.

And, not matter what anyone else may tell you, it's completely acceptable to ask around about someone's character within the age play or BDSM community. You can ask exes and former lovers for their opinion, but still take it with a grain of salt. You can even borrow a page from the escorting industry and verify someone's employment before you agree to meet them. While you should be discreet, you can ask how long they've been working there and verify their legal name. Be sure to check that the business is indeed real, via Yelp and Google reviews, driving by the location, etc.

Do not count on self-defense classes to keep you safe. The dumbest thing you can do is overestimate yourself, and underestimate a person who may be trying to harm you. If you walk into a room with someone who is taller, heavier, stronger, and more skilled than you are, you're most likely going to lose that fight. In fact, it would be a miracle if you didn't. And if that other person is luring you into a situation that they have set up, if they're armed and expecting you, you're probably not going to be able to get away from them. Remember that Neal Falls, the West Virginia man who was finally killed by one of his victims as he attempted to kidnap her, may be linked to the disappearances of ten or more women who weren't so lucky. You don't have to be afraid of everyone; just be smart!

Flagging

When moving about in groups that are aware of age play, you can flag, i.e. wear a certain item to let people know what sort of play you're interested in, what type of partner you're looking for, or what you identify as. This practice is native to the BDSM and Leather communities, and has swelled to include age play. Keeping that in mind, most people flag everyday without realizing it, from wearing gendered clothing to buckling their belt a certain way.

You may be familiar with flagging as "the hanky code". I prefer not to use this term because flagging goes beyond hankies. Keys, hand-cuffs, wallet chains, hair bows, and more can be employed.

Most people don't flag these days, at least not in the traditional sense, and even people who are aware of the practice don't always know the significance of every single item. However, even if you're not sure what a hanky color or item means in itself, you can infer some meaning from its placement. Dominants, tops, and providers of play wear items on the left side of the body. Submissives, bot-toms, and receivers of play wear items on the right side.

Flagging items relevant to age play include:

- Diaper pins.

- Hairbows.

- Toy baby key rings.

Hanky colors relevant to age play acts and identities include:

- Brown: scat play.

- Hunter green: Daddy roleplay or identity.

- Mint green: Mommy roleplay or identity.

- Terry cloth: diaper play.

- Yellow: pee play.

You can also flag using the age play pride symbol, which is often re-produced as a literal flag as well as emblazoned on pins, shirts, and other wearable items. The symbol was created in 2002 and has been given to the public domain. A free collection of files containing different versions of the symbol is available at theghidrah.com/#Projects.

Another version of the pride flag was created in 2005 by an ABDL known as David. This flag has also been gifted to the public domain and free, downloadable files are available at abdlscandinavia.com/abdlflag. The creator invites you to "feel free to print it on coffee cups, include it in web pages, [and] decorate your neighborhood[.]"[11]

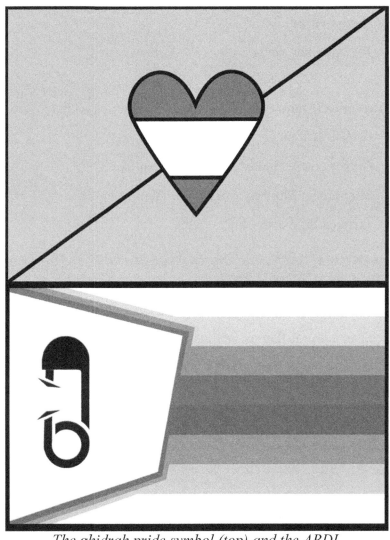

*The ghidrah pride symbol (top) and the ABDL
Scandinavia version (bottom). Littles Pride Day is
April 23.*

Flagging is especially useful in settings where people are aware of age play, but perhaps can't have completely blunt conversations about it. Two good examples would be munches and classes.

Munches

A munch is an informal meeting of people out in the vanilla, non-age play, non-kinky world. They usually take place once a month. Hopefully you live in an area that hosts a Littles munch, which you can probably find at littlesmunch.com. Like this book, munches may be directed at Littles, but everyone with an interest in age play is welcome. Munches provide a platform for new players to introduce themselves to veterans of the scene without the pressure or uncertainty that might exist at a play party. It's sort of a rehearsal.

Keep in mind that it's unlikely to be a *dress* rehearsal. Most munches take place at regular restaurants and coffee shops and have a casual, streetwear dress code. If you show up in a frilly, pink satin dress that shows your diaper, you will probably be asked to leave. When you wear fetish attire to a public meeting like that, you're not only making the vanilla people around you uncomfortable, you're essentially outing everyone at the munch as an age player without their consent. Save your over-the-top outfits and behavior for parties and events.

Talkative individuals should be mindful of not dominating the conversation. If you feel that you might be doing this, ask a question! Better yet, find someone who has been more quiet and ask *them* a question or two. There's no reason not to stand up and go over to someone to try to start a conversation. At the same time, try to be mindful of the fact that you're in a vanilla setting. Lower your voice when appropriate and try to speak in anagrams if possible. "Are you more of an AB or a DL?" is more discreet than the unabbreviated version.

If you have questions about the environment, group, and what's acceptable, you should be able to find some contact information for the organizer of the munch either on fetlife.com or on littesmunch.com. A good organizer will be friendly and forthcoming with information, but of course be polite and attempt to answer questions on your own before putting them out. Most organizers will provide a moderately discreet way to identify the group, such as placing a stuffed animal on their table. If you're not sure that you see the munch group, you can approach any group or another individual who appears to be waiting and simply ask, "Are you here for the munch?" If they ask for clarification, you know you're with the wrong people!

If you want to organize a munch, ask yourself the following questions:

- Would this munch be filling a void not otherwise met by another munch?

- Are there enough age players in my area to support a recurring, informal monthly meetup? Is my community not only stable, but growing?
- Am I well-known and well-liked enough in my group that people will support my munch with real-world actions and spending power?
- Can I find a location to host the munch that is inexpensive, accessible by public transit, accessible to those with disabilities, able to seat a large group of people, and tolerant of discussions of an adult nature at a reasonable, yet clearly audible volume? (Coffee shops and cafés are well-suited to these intersections of functions, so long as they aren't too cramped.)
- Can I commit to a monthly schedule?
- Am I good at breaking the ice and facilitating conversations between strangers?
- Am I good at arbitrating disputes? Could I deal with or expel an unruly, intoxicated, or otherwise inappropriate person with grace and civility?
- Am I ready to serve my Littles community and do I have the necessary promotional skills and online presence to do so?

Hopefully you answer yes to all of these questions before you start a local munch. Try to find an opportunity to attend another munch, possibly one that isn't age play-related or that isn't local, in order to gauge how they work, what is done, and what (if anything) could be improved. It's always better to support established community efforts rather than starting your own just because you want to be the leader.

Classes

Going out to classes is a great way to grow as an age player and even as a person. Unlike a play party or event, however, many people there may not be interested in meeting play partners or even making friends. I find that whenever I go to classes, there's always one person who tries to force a conversation with someone who is clearly not interested. It's typically a guy I've never seen before and I know that I'll never see him again. Don't be a cruiser. Come to classes to learn. You can also come to gauge your interest in attending actual events. After all, classes are often held in the same spaces in which people hold events and are often taught by the same people who host. You can grab a few flyers on your way out.

If you can't find an age play-specific class, look for some classes with crossover interest, like spanking or humiliation. You can even go for classes on more generic topics, like female domination. Feel free to ask a few questions that are specific to age play, but be respectful of others and don't try to turn the class into a personal consultation for yourself.

Most people attend classes in their street clothes and, if you're one of the cool kids, I suggest doing the same. Yes, there may be someone there in full fetish attire, but they look a little dorky. I taught one class where a woman showed up in street clothes only to change into a latex bodysuit in the bathroom. It seemed odd to me that she would change just to sit in a chair for an hour and a half and I had to wonder if she was having some sort of sexual experience while the rest of the attendees were just trying to learn. She seemed pretty uncomfortable and spent most of the class shifting in and squeaking her chair. I hope it was worth it: she probably had to go home and hand-wash that whole bodysuit!

The exception to this rule is classes that are offered as a part of a convention. You might be running to a play party right after the class and don't want to stop in at your hotel room or perhaps you want to give your clothes a little time to settle. Many people at a convention will be wearing some form of fetish attire for the entire weekend-long event, perhaps covering up in the common areas when appropriate.

I like to bring a notebook and pen with me to classes. Most people don't and you may feel a little nerdy, but if I'm taking time out of my day and paying money to learn something, I want to be sure to learn it. I also try to think specifically of what questions I want answered in the class and will have them written down. They're usually answered in the course of the lecture, but I can always raise my hand or speak to the presenter during the break or after the class if necessary.

Some class presenters will make time for questions. Others won't. Rain DeGrey uses a system that I've since adopted myself: she brings index cards and pens and invites class goers to write out their questions and deposit them into a vase during the break. That way she makes sure that everyone gets what they came to the class for and people can even maintain their anonymity if they're shy.

Pricing for classes varies. Some of them are free. Some of them cost hundreds or even thousands of dollars. Whatever the cost, remember that the person you're interacting with may, in fact, be a volunteer. Be respectful and thankful at all times. If the class is offered on a sliding scale, do pay the most that you possibly can. Remember that presenters must pay for materials out of pocket, locations need to pay their rent, and the knowledge that you're gaining is indeed valuable.

Play Parties

Littles parties may be hosted at a local playspace (which may or may not have a dungeon-aesthetic) or perhaps in someone's private residence. They usually come in two varieties: dark and light. At a dark age play party, which is usually held later in the day, people are expected to be more sexual and possibly to engage in BDSM or domestic discipline scenes. At a light age play party, which is usually held in the afternoon, there's usually a no sex rule or sex is only allowed in a particular area. I would say that there's sometimes a no kink rule, too, but adults running around in diapers and onesies and calling each other "Mommy", "Daddy," or what have you is probably pretty kinky to most people in the world. So it's more that the only kink allowed is age play and roleplay. Even spanking may be considered taking things too far. Try to see what other people are doing or just go ahead and ask if you want to do something that might be against the rules.

Most parties have a small fee associated with them. Remember that the host may have to pay rent to the hosting location, buy food and decorations, and more. When I attend parties, I often bring my adult-size rocking horse, which can necessitate the rental of a truck. If you really can't contribute financially, see if you can contribute by volunteering to act as a cashier or dungeon monitor. Special training is required for these positions, but you can sometimes also volunteer to help clean up or prepare snacks. If you can contribute financially, keep these positions free for others who may be more strapped for cash than you are.

It's usually completely acceptable to attend parties as a single person, and to wear age play clothes, though you may need to arrive in street clothes and change there. It's usually considered totally okay to wear and wet a diaper, but only if you do not leak on anything or cause an odor. You may need to change yourself in the bathroom, but there are often bondage tables, beds, and other surfaces suitable to changing a diaper which you can use so long as you use a changing pad and clean up after yourself. Many parties will be stocked with safer sex and other dungeon supplies, which include disposable chux, which are kind of like square, tapeless diapers that people use to prevent contamination of surfaces. They can be used in place of a changing pad, perhaps on top of a towel, which are often provided as well.

It is usually not considered okay to mess your diaper, as there may not be a place to dispose of it. If you're unsure about rules, ask the host. Remember that others usually don't want to be exposed to your malodorous waste and, if you don't care about the feelings of the people around you, you are free to play alone in your own home. Attending community events is a privilege, not a right, and it can be revoked!

Party etiquette is pretty universal, but people sometimes still don't understand it. Most of the rules have to do with consent and cleanliness. Not abiding by them can get you permanently banned from all events. Before attending any sort of BDSM, age play, sex, or kink event, be sure that you have drilled the following into your head:

- Do not touch any person or their things without express permission. Permission to touch a toy is not permission to use it. Permission to hug someone is not permission to kiss them. Don't play that boundary game.

- Only "yes" means yes. Silence, a maybe, etc. all count as a "no."

- If people are having a scene, i.e. if they are playing together, do not interrupt them. You may watch and even talk quietly with another person, but they should be able to comfortably ignore you and not hear any of your comments. You should be out of their personal space. If they have to ask you to move or be quiet, you've already been rude.

- Do not discuss the play party with outsiders. Do not out anyone without their express permission. Be very careful and remember that others' livelihoods and families may be at stake.

- Photography is generally forbidden, except at special photography parties and, even there, you may be required to get permission before photographing specific people. In general, it's good to get into the habit of asking people if you may take their picture before doing so.

- Limit your time in the play area to 15 to 30 minutes if the party is busy. Do your aftercare back in the lounge area. Remember that these are semi-public spaces. If you want to treat an area like your personal playspace, build a personal playspace. Usually parties aren't too busy, though, and you can stay in the play area for as long as you like.

- Keep your noise to a reasonable volume. Don't scream or shout continually, though some noise is expected and tolerated.
- Drugs and alcohol may not be permitted at all or may only be allowed in moderation. Sometimes this has to do with a space's insurance policy. At other events, alcohol use is encouraged.
- If you commit a faux pas or outright break a rule, accept correction gracefully and, if you can, try to make it right.

We live in a culture that doesn't normalize consent, which can make people feel more awkward obtaining it than they feel about violating it, which is, well, terrible. However, it isn't actually all that odd to obtain consent and people in the age play community will appreciate your doing so. That said, don't just walk up to everyone at a party and say, "Can I change your diaper?"

Consent rules are not a magical series of social moves that make people want to play with you. They're a way to make sure that people feel respected and secure enough to say no, which is good! Take the time to get to know people just for the sake of getting to know them and then, if you feel a connection and think that they might, too, you can tell them, "I'd love to take you over to that chair and give you a spanking, if you're game." Then negotiate their limits, safeword, and other concerns and opportunities.

If someone is overstepping your boundaries in any way, possibly by trying to pressure you into play (i.e. aggressively cruising), touching you without your permission, or telling you that you have to call them by a certain title, you can let a dungeon monitor or even the party organizer know. You don't have to put up with that. You can be discreet about it if you're feeling shy.

Once, at a fetish convention, I saw a young woman approach a security guard and explain to him that a man had been following her and was becoming increasingly threatening when she declined his advances. She described this man in detail, including his unusual outfit and gold tooth. The security guard argued that the man was simply exercising free speech and that there was nothing that he could do about it. I marched over there and informed him that she had a right to go about her day unmolested and that it was his job as a security officer to make sure that people at this private event were safe. The officer continued to argue, unaware that I knew the event organizer and had worked with her on several occasions. I texted her about the issue immediately. If a staff member at a party refuses to help you, go over their head. If you see someone's concerns being ignored, step in and try to help. If you're working security, do your job and help to keep people safe.

Beyond personal safety and consent, let's talk about cleanliness. Most spaces will be equipped with cleaning and personal health supplies, like condoms and extra sheets. I recommend checking in with a dungeon monitor or other volunteer if you're new to a space and need help navigating their cleaning protocol. Below is an outline of basic cleaning protocol.

- If you are playing on a surface, especially in a state of undress, put down a towel, sheet, or disposable chux underpad. Towels and sheets are more for basic play where someone might just get a little sweaty. Chux are for play that will involve bodily fluids, like a diaper change or sex.
- When you are done playing, put towels and sheets into the hamper. Throw away soiled chux.
- Wipe down surfaces before disinfecting with a paper towel and some alcohol, bleach, or "toy cleaner" (usually antibacterial soap and water which has been mixed in a spray bottle) to cut surface grease and dirt.
- After the surface has been wiped down, spray it with a disinfectant. Some spaces will have hospital-grade cleaners like MadaCide-1, or you may just have to use alcohol or bleach again. Leave the disinfectant on the surface for at least ten

minutes before wiping up.

- Put all your cleaning items away when you're done.

If you're bringing your own toys and items with play with, don't forget to clean them, too, before you put them back in your toy bag. You may want to bring zip-top bags, leather wipes, or other cleaning items to care for your own things. It is generally acceptable to use the venue's items to clean your personal belongings. However, it is not considered polite to clean soiled sex toys in the venue's sink. Instead, put them in a plastic bin or bag and take them home to be cleaned.

If you're hosting a party for the first time, I trust that you know people in your community, are ready for the financial burden of doing so, and have attended and volunteered at other parties in order to prepare yourself.

First, decide what type of party you want and pick a suitable locale. Are you prepared to pay for a hotel suite? Are you prepared to tone down behavior in a free, public setting? Are you prepared to dedicate at least an hour to set up and another hour to clean up at a dungeon space? Are you able to decorate a space? Is your location accessible to those with disabilities?

Littles parties work best, I find, with a theme and set activities, while still allowing time and space for people to do their own thing. Just setting up and letting people do whatever works okay, but don't expect an epic party. I used to think that play parties were really just open spaces for people to explore on their own, but I admit that I was wrong. It's better to think of them as regular parties and plan for things like ice breaker games.

Try to find a theme that resonates with your local community. I've had good luck with the themes summer camp, fairy tales, Halloween, school, etc. Your theme should be self-explanatory, conjure up strong imagery, and be inclusive. For example, "Boy Scouts" may sound like a fun theme, but just "Scouts" will get more people people to attend and there won't be confusion as to whether the event is just for men. (Don't count on people clicking on your event link to learn that, no, in fact all genders are welcome when the very title excludes them.) The theme can also help to dictate activities.

Activities should be accessible to everyone, including people with disabilities. If you overlooked someone and notice that they aren't able to participate, try to discreetly see if there's something else that they would like to do. If they're happy to just watch, be sure to be friendly and inclusive toward them anyway.

There are many great books of children's party games that will give you ideas--and most of those games are inexpensive or even free to put together. I recommend *Hopscotch, Hangman, Hot Potato, and Ha, Ha, Ha: a Rulebook of Children's Games* by Jack Maguire. The games are simple, fun, don't require much preparation, and are organized according to a variety of environmental situations. Some activities can be assembled at the party as a craft, like making a bowling set out of soda bottles or a fort out of cardboard. While games can be sexualized, I recommend against it in a party where people might not all know each other and it's out of the question for a light age play party. Party games for teenagers, like Suck and Blow or Spin the Bottle which are lightly sexual might work okay for dark age play parties. Small prizes from the dollar store can add to the fun.

If you're providing food at your event, you may want to use your event description to invite people to notify you of food allergies. It's good to have nut-free and vegetarian options--in fact, I think you'd have to be trying not to. Anything that does contain nuts or meat but may not appear to should be labeled.

Age play parties can get to be expensive. If you're having trouble affording them, look into funding options like charging for admittance or asking for a donation, perhaps on a sliding scale. Consider raffling off some donated or homemade items. You can also look into free resources, like your local library, which is truly a great resource for age play parties. There are science project kits, juvenile soundtracks, kids' movies, and, of course, books for storytime or of game ideas.

You can mention to your community if you're having a hard time coming up with the money, but don't leave it at that. Instead, have a list of what you actually need, like snacks, a sound system, a location, or games. That way you'll be inviting people to help you rather than just complaining or panhandling. In fact, you'll be community-building, which is what parties are ultimately all about!

If your local Littles community is small or you don't have the time or resources to plan a full party, you can organize a takeover or a Littles corner of a party in your local Leather community instead. A takeover is when a group of people, Littles in this case, all attend an event en masse and simply make a point of having a presence there. Just announce the takeover to your fellow age players after clearing it with the host.

A Littles corner is pretty much what it sounds like. It's a small space that has been equipped for age players to have an accommodating niche at a BDSM play party. If you're setting up a Littles corner, bring some age play accoutrements with you, like coloring books and crayons, play dough, blocks, etc. Coordinate with the host before you announce your Littles corner. In fact, the host will probably mention that the party has a Littles corner in their promotional copy.

Outings

Some age play groups host public outings. I'm lucky to live in San Francisco, which is basically age play heaven and offers a number of locales that make for amazing age play outings, from museums and zoos to specialty ice cream bars and night clubs.

If you don't live in an area with as many public places that seem almost designed with age play in mind, there's nothing wrong with a good, old fashioned park. Of course age playing in public requires more discretion. You don't want to be arrested for public indecency after a diaper change. You also don't want to force a parent to have a conversation with a child that the child isn't ready for. Just because you *can* do something doesn't mean that you *should*. Keep your actions discreet and be considerate when you're on an age play outing.

Also keep in mind that certain public areas are more accepting of unusual behavior from adults. If you're organizing an outing, try to find a location that isn't over populated by real children. I've found that areas populated by tourists also work well. Yes, there may be chronological children there, but they usually expect to see some odd stuff--at least in a major metropolitan area. The trade off is that they may feel free to photograph you without your permission.

When the lovely Siouxsie Q was planning her age play birthday party, she had the idea to reserve a section of a local park. She even went so far as to get a permit for a bouncy house! The result was a semi-private location where we could get into our Little headspace while still running about and not feeling cooped up. It was pretty cool--until, I kid you not, a bus of tourists showed up. Luckily things were mostly over by then, but it just goes to show that, no matter how well prepared you are, you can always be thrown a curveball!

Groups

Little Scouts If you're looking for friends and a sense of community, Little Scouts may be for you! The Little Scouts are an 18-and-over, inclusive age play scout troop dedicated to spreading awareness of age play and providing community for Littles without Bigs. They go on trips, earn badges, volunteer, and do all sorts of things for their local communities.

There are several Little Scout troops across America and you can easily set up your own chapter. Each chapter is completely independent and makes up its own rules, badge criteria, etc. so you can pretty much do what you like. Some chapters only have sashes while others have entire uniforms! thelittlescouts.com

Skipping Club Vanilla age players have gotten pretty bold lately. In

2015 in New York, a woman named Michelle Joni even started Preschool Mastermind, a preschool for adults which took place on Tuesday evenings in March, from 7:00 pm to 10:00 pm. Joni is also the brains behind Skipping Club which is, well, what it sounds like, and many other free-spirited events. michellejoni.com or skippingclub.com

Muir Academy Established in 1987, the Muir Academy is located in Wye Valley in Wales. The Academy promotes itself as "the perfect place to indulge your adult school roleplay fantasies." They even have a set uniform and application process. muir-academy.co.uk

New Grange Manor New Grange Manor, also located in the United Kingdom, offers an immersive school roleplay experience in the same manner as Muir Academy. While you have to be over 21 years of age to attend the Academy, you only have to be 18 to attend the Manor. The Manor offers not only a special uniform and application process, but four different Houses, a la Harry Potter! You can be sorted into the Celts, Romans, Saxons, or Vikings. Younger age players can enroll in their preschool. ngmanor.co.uk

Conventions

A convention is sort of like an extended, open age play party, peppered with munches and classes. You'll be able to learn, shop, play, and mingle, as you like. There seem to be more and more such events every year. While there are conventions specific to age play, age players are welcome at a plethora of conventions, ranging in focus from BDSM to furries. It's normal for exact locations to be kept secret until after you've paid for your ticket, though you should be told the general location upfront.

When someone says "convention" most people probably think of a large, multiple-day gathering that takes place in a hotel. However, lots of age players are arranging age play camping trips, such as the amusingly-named Dipstock (fetlife.com/groups/119530), which are basically outdoor conventions, perhaps with less emphasis on education and shopping. These types of events are common also in the BDSM community and there is some crossover at events like Camp Crucible.

There are also some non-kink, adult events like Camp Grounded (campgrounded.org), Adult Music Camp (adultmusiccamp.com), and Soul Camp (soul.camp), to name a few. These camps are openly described as "summer camp for adults", though most of the attendees likely have no idea what age play is or that they're engaging in it. Other such events might include gaming, toy, and comic book conventions, though these are adult-focused rather than adults-only.

Vanilla events like these can certainly be fulfilling to your Little, but are not the place to fly your age play pride flag, if you get my drift, especially if you don't want to give your fellow age players a bad name. Attend and have a lovely time, but be considerate and extra discreet! Yes, the guy next to you may be making a lanyard, but he probably doesn't want to hear about how you're going to give yours to your Mommy.

Here's a list of current conventions that are welcoming of or focused on age players:

Camp Abdulia Camp Abdulia is "mostly a party to meet other ABDLs and the curious and socialize...at night, we let our hair down and get a little wild."[12] There are a few misconceptions about Camp Abdulia, namely that only younger people are allowed to attend. This apparently isn't true, though their FetLife group does say, "Camp Abdulia is a private party held for the younger generation of ABDLs & Ageplayers." Since you have to be pre-approved in order to attend, you'll be able to double check. fetlife.com/groups/58125

Camp Crucible Though not specifically an age play event, this epic nine-day and eight-night event has a very, very strong age play presence. Located on the east coast, this BDSM camp supports a Kidz Camp where age players can bunk together and immerse themselves in 24/7 age play! campcrucible.com

CAPCon Short for Chicago Age Players Convention, CAPCon is an age play-specific gathering. Besides classes and activities, CAPCon organizers go above and beyond to construct age play areas that include things like cubbies and changing stations. chicagoageplayers.com

TeddyCon This Pennsylvania convention promises a fun-filled weekend for age players and their partners that includes crafts, classes, movie time, and more! They are equipped with special age play furniture and toys and have even managed to attract corporate sponsors, special guests, and age play-specific vendors! teddycon.org

US Littles This convention, based in Montana, promotes itself as a sort of world summit on age play and diaper fetishism. You need to be vetted by the event's organizers before you can attend. uslittles.com

If you're attending your first convention ever, or just attending a specific con for the first time, familiarize yourself with their official rules. Try to look around the con's website and find some pictures so that you'll get an idea of what everyone else will be wearing and doing. Go through their schedule and make sure there are events that you'll find engaging.

Don't show up expecting others to owe you any particular type of experience. You have to make your own. If someone declines to play with you, accept it gracefully and give them their space. Cruising for pick up play may be acceptable in one area, but not another. Try to "read the air" and see how others are behaving before you dive in, while keeping in mind that the person you're watching may be super popular due to years of volunteering and organizing--or maybe they just know everyone. Take the time to make friends and try to add something to the event. Don't force it and, if someone seems disinterested, happily give them their space.

When reading through the convention's rules or code of conduct, you should know that some rules exist to protect the con organizers from legal ramifications, some exist to ensure that outsiders are not offended, some exist to protect the convention's location and its owners, and some exist to create a certain vibe. You must obey them all, whether or not you agree with them. Even if you can do whatever you like in the conference rooms, many cons have special rules about behavior in the host hotel's common areas which may include vanilla dress codes. If you want the con to continue to run and be welcome at their host hotel, err on the side of not offending staff members and other guests. Think about what may be offensive to the staff, rather than what you find offensive. Even something as simple as a pacifier in the mouth may be a step too far.

If you have any cool age play furniture, you might want to offer to bring it to the con either for use at a specific event or to be left in a playroom for open play. Ask about their insurance policy and be sure that they'll look after your piece. You can also volunteer to help out, which will sometimes get you free admission or a reduced ticket price, just like at a play party.

When packing for a con, bring a variety of clothes, including regular street clothes and fetish clothes. Don't forget diapers and other fetish items, but pack them up discreetly. Most con hotels also have a pool or at least a hot tub, so you might want to bring something to swim in.

Professional Playmates

Yes, professional players are part of the community, too. Oftentimes we're the most involved because we literally make it our business to be! We have access to dungeons, training, and toys that the civilian population can only dream about, so don't feel weird about including us! We're useful allies and make great friends. (Note that being a friend doesn't mean getting free play or fetish attention. Quite the opposite: a friend is happy to support my business and won't ask for free labor!)

The perks of playing with a professional Mommy or Daddy (or auntie, uncle, teacher, nurse, Little, babysitter, or whatever) are increased privacy and a drastically increased chance of play. I say the chance of play is increased rather than guaranteed because very bad behavior can get you banned, usually without a refund, by the way. Of course, as a sex worker, I'm biased towards thinking that we're a great solution to the issue of un-partnered, eager players. I've had some amazing experiences with my professional playmates, learned new skills, and gotten some great stories. My clients have often seemed to enjoy their time with me as well, and in some cases, we've formed strong friendships.

If you're looking for a Mommy or Daddy, you can usually find a BDSM professional sex worker who offers age play sessions with relative ease, so long as you live in or travel to a city of notable size. There are a number of sites that list sex workers who specialize in BDSM, domestic discipline, and fetishes. Good places to start include eros-guide.com and maxfisch.com. It can be more difficult to find a Little (or any type of submissive), but it is still possible.

Before you contact a sex worker, take the time to sift through their online presence. It's considered rude in the digital age to ask for information that is readily accessible and it makes you look like a rube to do so. You don't want to get a bad reputation and sex workers talk to each other. Have the following information ready before you attempt to book someone:

- A basic outline of what you would like to happen, in keeping with the sex worker's limitations, which should be listed on their website. If you can't come up with such an outline, you're not ready to see a sex worker. Keep in mind that "sex worker" is a blanket term for people who provide sex in all its forms, and penis in vagina (PIV) penetration may be off the menu or they may not offer any sexual contact at all, only fantasy scenarios.

- Your availability. Be specific, but also offer a range. I don't recommend asking for the sex worker's availability, because it changes as they accept bookings. In the time that you write back, someone else may have offered them a session instead of adding that extra step! If your schedule is very open, just say so, but in my experience when a client says this, their schedule isn't really as open as they claim and they probably should have just pitched a date.

- How long you would like to session for. I find that one to two hours is good for a first session. Do not expect that time will be kept free for you to extend, but you can always mention that you may want to extend the session. This may or may not change how your session or others are booked. Only ask about extensions if you really mean it!

- Your relevant limits. I often get people telling me "no necrophilia." Do they really think that I'm going to randomly start pretending to be dead in the middle of an ABDL session? If you're unsure of your limits, just think of things that might happen that would be problematic. Do you want a spanking, but not marks? Do you want to wet, but not mess? Do you enjoy enemas, but not suppositories? Be clear!

- If you would like an incall or an outcall location for the session. If you are requesting an outcall location, you need to let them know where it is, at least approximately.

Don't ask a sex worker to reassure you that they're into your fetish. If they offer a type of play, they enjoy it. People don't last long doing sex work that they don't like. If you're really worried about this, go with someone who has at least five years of professional experience.

Do not ask for a play-by-play of what will happen in session; this is just asking for cyber sex, whether you mean to or not. While the sex worker will take the reins once you arrive, it is up to you to communicate your needs and desires outside of session. Don't fall back on, "I want whatever you want," unless you're into hardcore financial domination!

If, by some chance, you have a terrible session, handle it with dignity. Try communicating. Leave early if you have to and be polite. You might say something like, "I feel like we're not communicating well and I think that I'm just going to call it a day." Again, you don't want a bad reputation, but you also don't have to hang around.

If the sex worker is willing to give a full or partial refund, they will offer it, but it isn't likely. They may need to cover costs like childcare, equipment, travel, space rental, etc. Remember that from where they're sitting, you may just not have the necessary negotiation skills and be wasting their time. I've only once had someone break down in session and I feel that it was due to his own poor negotiation and unrealistic expectations of himself. I was happy to help him through those issues and we had subsequent sessions, but I wasn't about to offer a refund.

Some websites give you the option to write a review. Many sex workers don't even like positive reviews, because they can be admitted as evidence in court--and not necessarily a criminal trial, but, say, a child custody hearing. If they ask you to leave one or say that they don't mind, remember that if you can't say something nice, you shouldn't say anything at all. Instead of seeking the emotional satisfaction that you might get from leaving a negative review, go see someone who is better suited to your desires. At the very least, you now have a sex worker who can provide a reference for you as being a safe, polite client. Be as professional and considerate as you would want the sex worker to be.

If you're thinking about becoming a sex worker, know that it is indeed work. There is money there, but it isn't easy money. Ofelia del Corazon wrote an article titled *10 Tips for the Aspiring Feminist Dominatrix*, which I suggest that you read. I also recommend *Lessons I Learned as a Dominatrix: 10 Things That Don't Exist* by Mitsu. To become a sex worker, either in the real world or via webcam, you will need to:

- Take classes.
- Attend events.
- Maintain an online presence on relevant forums.
- Pay for advertising.
- Build and maintain a website.
- Keep up on trends in sexuality and advertising.
- Find and read or view porn for session ideas, but take them with a grain of salt and think about how these things would work in reality.
- Answer countless emails, many of which will not result in a booking. (I counter this by charging an application fee on niteflirt.com, which takes a percentage, but results in a 99% booking rate by ensuring that my applicants are serious.)
- Buy and maintain a wardrobe.
- Find and hire a professional photographer.
- Learn to use Photoshop or hire a graphic designer.
- Find and rent a pre-existing playspace or orchestrate your

own.

- Connect with other local sex workers in order to learn the slang, get "doubles" bookings and receive training on things like safety, billing, and sanitation. You probably can't find a mentor without at least one year of experience under your belt. We like to know that you're serious. Even then it's hard, but keep an eye out. My mentor is Natasha Strange of kittenwithawhip.com and her advice and training have been invaluable both in and out of the dungeon.
- Take classes on makeup application so that you will look gorgeous without looking made up or develop a signature makeup style.
- Buy makeup and supplies.
- Keep financial records up to date.

These things are the bare minimum. Why? Because everyone you're competing with does these things. If you want to excel, you'll need to do more, like teaching, writing, and traveling. I feel that I should also mention that unless you also have a day job, you will have trouble applying for loans, renting a living space, and making other financial moves. You may not be able to use PayPal, Square, or other online payment processors, as they often ban users who are known sex workers,[13] like yours truly, even if we're only making completely innocent transactions. (They keep the money when they do that, by the way.) There is also special discrimination against age play sex workers within the adult industry. For example, you will not be able to use CC Bill, the biggest, best adult payment processor around.[14]

As for the literal payoff, your rates should be the cost of your playspace multiplied by four if you do not have sex with your clients and the same as the average local lawyer's hourly rate if you do, perhaps plus the cost of your playspace. I recommend that you take the time to read *Beat the Heat: How to Handle Encounters with Law Enforcement* by Katya Komisaruk if you are any type of sex worker. You should also have the number of a local lawyer who specializes in sex workers' rights. Try to obtain a copy of the *St. James Infirmary Occupational Health & Safety Handbook* and peruse it. You can also find the *Handbook* in PDF form online at stjamesinfirmary.org. Find the websites for your local advocacy groups--and have a backup plan for if they fail you. Because there's so much variance, it's important to be familiar with the laws, conventions, and resources in your immediate area.

These are just the basics to try to make sure that you stay safe and are competitive and lucrative. If you would like more information or a better idea of what to expect from clients, try reading *Paying for It: a Guide by Sex Workers for Their Clients*, edited by Greta Christina. It's a good starting place and a variety of types of sex workers contributed to it, giving you a wide range of experience and covering a myriad of topics.

Being a sex worker is often extremely difficult, but it's also extremely rewarding. Sometimes I feel like you have to do the boring, hard parts for free and get paid well for the fun, exciting parts. You get to meet and play with interesting, enthusiastic people that you otherwise wouldn't be able to fit into your schedule and you are regularly exposed to play scenarios that otherwise might not have been options for you. My favorite part is crafting elaborate, fulfilling scenes and seeing my client's eyes light up as his fantasy comes to life around him. (And, in case you were wondering, no: you will not really be getting any women as clients. I've had three in ten years and they all came with their husbands. Men hoping to get women as clients: don't hold your breath.)

Fostering Acceptance

Most larger kink communities are open to age play and welcome age players warmly. If you find yourself in a community that isn't open to age play, don't despair. There are things that you can do to facilitate acceptance. No, you shouldn't *have* to, but the reality is that sometimes you do.

In the event of ongoing intolerant behavior, try arranging a meeting with your local community leaders. First, email them about the issues you've been having and ask them if they can think of why others might be having a hard time acclimating to your presence. This will give you an idea of which specific obstacles you can help them overcome. Then, ask them to meet with you either at a neutral location or at the local dungeon, not during a play party, but just to talk. Put together an agenda of points to discuss and have materials on hand to help you.

It's also important to have a clear idea of an implementable solution to the problem. If you just want to vent, do it to your diary. Examples of good solutions include:

- Having a Littles corner set up at at least six play parties per year.
- Training staff and volunteers to be supportive of Littles and to moderate disputes with other players who may question their right to share the space.
- Raising funds to bring out an educator to teach a class on age play or, more broadly, on taboo roleplay.
- Arranging to have more age play-friendly dungeon furniture brought in, like a rocking horse or a massage table that can double as a changing table.

Hopefully your community leaders will be reasonable and helpful. From there, it's up to you to continue to attend events in Little mode in order to facilitate conversations and to show that age play accept-

ance is a real concern, even if only for your Little ol' self. Ultimately, it is the responsibility of the people who are being unaccept-
ing to alter their own behavior, but since you can only control yourself, you might as well try to lead them in the right direction and en-
list help where you can.

If you are a community leader reading this looking for better ideas
of how you can help your local Littles community to feel more involved and accepted, thank you for being open-minded and taking a
proactive step in building a better Leather community. If you require
more help, tips, or suggestions for your specific community, you can
reach out to the Little Scouts at thelittlescouts.com. One of the aims
of the organization is to help in situations like these. They may be
able to offer advice or materials to assist you.

Coming Out

Coming out as an age player is not the same thing as coming out as
being gay or transgender or intersex. It's more like coming out as a
stocking fetishist or sharing who your favorite porn star is. Sure it's
part of who you are, but most people don't need to know about it. It
is still a coming out process, though.

Usually, the only reason to come out to someone you're not in a relationship with is to protect yourself in the event of a future outing

either by accident or a malicious party. You can do it arbitrarily or only when there's a creeping possibility of being outed. Either way, it's a risk and coming out as an age player to someone you're dependent on, be it a parent with whom you live or the person who signs your paychecks, is riskier still. If you feel the urge to come out to a friend, ask yourself if *they* would honestly feel that your relationship would be enhanced by knowing about your Little side, especially if they never interact with it. Have they shared private parts of their sexual identity with you? Would it make them uncomfortable?

If you're a very active Little who has established a place in the local community and regularly attends events, your age play habits and accouterments may be a more visible part of your life and briefly explaining them can help you to avoid a lot of possibly awkward white lies. On the other hand, white lies can protect you, your family, and your career. Just make sure that you keep them straight and have practiced them in advance.

Limited, honest explanations can be an effective substitute for a full coming out. For example, if someone finds your diapers and ask questions, you can just say, "I wear them sometimes," and that will usually preclude further questions, unless they're very rude. If they are very rude, you can simply tell them, "I don't want to talk about this. It's inappropriate and embarrassing. Let's go get ice cream instead," which is completely honest, yet doesn't really expose your Little or your fetish.

Rather than "coming out" to your partner, I like to think of it as introducing them to age play. I think it gives a more accurate idea of what's actually going on here. This can still go horribly wrong and you're taking a risk when you do it. There is no foolproof way to go about it. I do have to admit, however, that I was introduced by a partner and it went very well. It happened to synch up with the sexual interests that I had been too embarrassed to mention to my partner, which is a rare coincidence.

I also introduced my current partner and helped develop my submissive boy's interests. Both of these scenarios have gone pretty well! My partner is now my Daddy and diapers me on occasion and my boy enthusiastically enjoys his Little diaper time. Getting my boy into age play was actually the result of a misunderstanding: I thought that he was already into it and hence made some bold, overconfident moves very early on. Getting my partner into it, on the other hand, was very deliberate and took a number of gentle, exploratory conversations over a period of years.

There are two different approaches to consider when you're thinking of introducing a partner to age play: one big conversation or many small ones. They both have their merits and drawbacks, which may be better or worse depending on your unique situation. Proceed with caution! It's unlikely that you'll be able to consult with someone who knows your partner well, so you're going to have to trust your own judgement on this and take a chance.

Sitting your partner down for one, big, all out discussion is great because it allows you to select an environment conducive to a deep conversation and to have educational materials ready. It also allows your partner to know that they're having it all out. They don't have to worry as much about what you may reveal next.

The drawbacks to this approach are that it can be a lot to take in all at once. Should your partner feel pressured to give an answer as to whether or not they want to engage in your interests, it's sometimes much easier to just say no--or to say yes and not really mean it. Be sure that your partner knows that they can take some time to assimilate this new information before deciding what to do with it.

The second option is to address individual aspects of play as they come up organically. This is sort of what my ex-husband did with me and what I did with my current partner. It's nice because it allows you to have a number of smaller, less exhausting conversations over time, but also to address individual points more fully. It doesn't feel as overwhelming. However, it can leave your partner dreading what's coming next. Even if you start this way, you may need to sit down and have a more lengthy conversation, especially if they go poking about online, looking for more information, and find something concerning or that doesn't apply to you and your situation.

Conversations with my current partner more or less followed this progression:

1. I asked to call him Daddy during sex and he agreed, though he was surprised.

2. I mentioned that I used to engage in Daddy-daughter roleplay with my ex-husband and that, for me, this was an incarnation of BDSM that fulfilled my submissive side. We discussed the Daddy Dom/little girl dynamic.

3. We had the talk about how age play differs from pedophilia.

4. I mentioned that I liked wearing juvenile clothes during sex and pointed out the age play aesthetics that he enjoyed, like pigtails, ruffles, and bows.

5. I admitted that I was a diaper fetishist and, months later, he said that he was interested in diapering me. A couple of months after that, he did. (It was all very slow, but patience paid off!)

These conversations took place over three years, but they were always encouraging. I got through those three years by age playing on my own, making the most of my professional sessions, and blogging. It was worth it. I still don't get as much Little time as I might like, but I tell myself that longing builds character. The timeline was significantly sped up with my ex-husband, but he would stage events. For example, he set me up to find his stash of cloth diapers. He literally put them into the bottom of a box of lingerie and then handed it to me to go through. I've gotta admit that it worked, but I'm pretty open minded and your mileage may vary.

No matter which method you choose, it's best to have a confident demeanor. Don't go into the conversation acting suspicious, creepy, or embarrassed. You're sharing a wonderful, powerful secret that will potentially bring you and your partner closer together. Make it clear to your partner that you're happy to answer any questions and that you will respect their decisions as to whether or not to participate.

Your partner may make a connection between age play and pedophilia. Be prepared for this event, which is unfortunately common. Remind them that you are both adults and that you are only getting older. Show them that age play events and online communities are for adults only. Make it clear that you're only interested in adults. I like to show partners an image that I found years ago and don't have the permission to reproduce here. It shows a buxom, adult woman stuffed into a crib, her limbs draped over the edges, an uncertain look in her eyes, various trappings of the nursery scattered about, and a tiny bib clasped around her neck. Despite her childish situation, she looks very adult. In fact, it makes her look even more adult.

Explaining the desire to age play is becoming easier and easier. Most of us in our majority now grew up with Nickelodeon kid power and that Toys "R" Us mentality of "I don't wanna grow up!" There are vanilla summer camps for adults now and, for a while, three of the ten best-selling books on Amazon were coloring books for grown ups.[15] Age play just takes it to a new level involving not only indulgence, but a loss of control, increased intimacy, and innocent security.

If your partner is okay with your Little side, but doesn't want to play with you, you should still count yourself lucky. Even if you don't want to continue the relationship with someone who isn't interested in playing with you, that kind of acceptance is not something you'll encounter everyday. If you do want to stay with your partner, you might want to discuss which ways you can still get your Little time. And, of course, do your best to leave the door open for future play should your partner change their mind.

You and your partner may decide to end the relationship over your revelation. Your partner may also decide to expose you to your friends, family, workplace, and community. Hopefully they have more grace than that, but it can happen and may adversely affect you. This is why it may be a good idea to have a contingency plan and can be a good idea to have prepared your loved ones, peers, and coworkers for the knowledge that you engage in an alternative lifestyle, even if you don't get specific. Most people will understand the difference between *private* and *secret* and will respect both your right to privacy and your right to live as you like.[16]

When having these difficult conversations, remember to stay calm and try not to get emotional. Really listen to the other person's concerns so that you can address them well. Realize that they may just need time and be ready to give it to them. Rather than forcing them to have a conversation they're not ready for or into saying something they'll regret, give them a little space, say for a week or a month or longer, and then come back and try for acceptance again.

Only you can decide if it's time share your Little side with someone. It isn't something that you can undo, so be very careful and keep those fingers crossed!

Subcultures

There are numerous age play subcultures, which seems only natural as age play mixes so well with other types of play. Here I've tried to create a list of subcultures that share aesthetics, behaviors, and fetishes. I decided not to include subcultures that have developed surrounding certain dynamics, like Daddy Dom/little girl (DD/lg).

The reason for this is that there aren't necessarily sizeable groups surrounding every single dynamic, and I don't want to reinforce stereotypes. Just because the Daddy Dom/little girl community has developed a strong presence doesn't mean that Mommy Dom/little boy couples don't exist. Anyway, such an exhaustive list would be obnoxiously long, especially considering polyamorous and switch relationships. I decided not to include groups based on sexual orientation for the same reason.

Babyfurs Babyfurs are the age play contingent of the furries, a fandom that centers around anthropomorphic creatures which may or may not actually have fur. Catgirls and other pet players are generally considered to be distinct from the furry community.

The babyfurs are an unexpectedly strong subculture, even having developed their own slang. "Cubbing out" is age playing as a babyfur while "getting padded" refers to regressing while diapered. Their entry on wikifur.com is extensive, including a history of the babyfur community dating back to 1995, a list of notable babyfurs, and the discrepant viewpoints that grow up within any sizeable community.[17]

Babyfurs can have one or more personas, just like any age player or furry. These personas are commonly expressed through real life or online roleplay, wearing fursuits, or drawing or commissioning art. The babyfur persona may or may not be expressed specifically for sexual reasons. They may be of any sexual orientation, including asexual. They run the full gamut of humanity, just like anyone.

Note that the term "anthro" (as in "anthropomorphic") may be more aptly applied to certain individuals who may at first appear to be furries. Some people prefer it partly because it lacks the stigma of the term "furry". It is also innately more inclusive of characters who may have scales or feathers instead of fur. However, "anthro" isn't just the politically correct term for a furry. There are subtle differences. An anthro's physique is generally closer to that of an animal and clothes are not worn. The character retains full animal instincts and human intelligence.

BDSM, Kink, & Leather What I will collectively call the Leather community has become much more accepting of age players in recent years. This welcoming attitude wasn't always the norm. In the past it wasn't unusual for age players to be asked to leave parties. A few problematic players certainly contributed to negative stereotypes, but our communal good will and efforts have, in the end, paid off! We're being catered to with hosted events, Littles Corners, title contests, and other daily forms of recognition.

BDSM lends itself well to the inherent power dynamics involved with many age play scenarios. The Kink community seems to empathize with a harmless behavior that nevertheless seems to lead to the discomfort of others. Leather culture embraces age play as an expression of an alternative lifestyle or sexuality. It was really only a matter of time before age players integrated with and grew up inside of these communities. And I'm glad we finally did. We all have a lot to offer one another!

Dark Age Play The dark age play subculture focuses on incorporating sex, or at least more conventionally recognized sex, with age play. While age players who may not strongly identify as dark age players may engage in overt, subtle, or even clandestine sexual activity, dark age players more directly enjoy the crossover of sexuality and regressive play.

Alternately, the term "dark age play" can mean play which incorporates classic BDSM. It can also refer to age play that focuses on role-playing darker themes, like molestation, incest, and domestic violence. This is why some people consider dark age play to be "edge play", which is a subjective term applied to play that people may consider to be especially subversive or dangerous.

Of course, some people consider all age play to be edge play, whether dark or light. Susan Wright organized the first age play titleholder contest, Little Miss & Mister Little, in 2009. During a 2014 interview, she told me how she first learned about age play and how it was perceived in her local Leather community.

> *I would watch Lolita Wolf, a good friend in New York City, age play at events. I was fascinated by the reaction to her. There would be all this really extreme stuff going on, but a girl sitting in a dress, coloring, was freaking people out. I thought it was really cool.*

> *This was back in 1991, '92, '93. Being a Little was considered to be inappropriate play in public, but people were doing it on their own, even though it's complete roleplay and there shouldn't be a problem with it.* [18]

I like to bring this up because some light age players can be a little snooty to dark age players. I like to remind them that not too long ago, all age players were subjected to that type of attitude. Yes, there are certain behaviors that people can engage in which are *not* acceptable, but when it comes to dark age play, as Miss Wright puts it, "there shouldn't be a problem with it."

Diaper Lovers Another subculture that sometimes squicks out age players are diaper fetishists, affectionately known as "diaper lovers" or "DLs". They aren't exactly a subset of age player, but there is a lot of crossover in paraphernalia and interests and they tend to move in the same circles. Of course, age play can squick out DLs, too. I suppose it all comes out in the wash.

At any rate, DLs are people who enjoy wearing diapers. DLs may just wear their diapers or they may wet, mess, or wet *and* mess them. Sometimes the fetish doesn't manifest sexually--or so I'm told. Every DL I've ever met who said that it wasn't sexual has turned out to be a sexual fetishist in the most traditional sense. I'm not sure if they just thought that telling me that it wasn't sexual would increase their chances of playing with me or that they didn't realize the true depths of their interests until they were able to indulge in them with another person or what--and thus far no one has been able to give me an answer. Still, I've heard the claim often enough to believe that it warranted a mention, and seen it turn out not to be true often enough that I thought I should mention that as well. If you are a DL who isn't aroused by diapers, good for you! We just haven't met yet.

Sissies Not all sissies are into age play or diapers, but there is a subset that is. Many sissy and crossdressing stores, such as birchplaceshop.com, stock adult baby-style clothes. In fact, visiting theadultbabystore.com will take you straight to Birch Place Shop's targeted splash page featuring adorable rompers, babydolls, diaper covers, bibs, bonnets, and more in a variety of fetish materials.

Sissy crossdressers are different from transgender women. Transgender women are women. Sissies are crossdressers. To clarify, a transgender woman may enjoy wearing over-the-top "sissy" styles either as a fashion statement or in the bedroom, but she isn't a crossdresser. I mean, I'm a cisgender woman and I have a few "sissy" items in my wardrobe as well. It was actually a bit of a joke at one of the dungeons I sessioned at for a while: a lot of my clothing overlapped with the sissy wardrobe. If you can't tell if someone is a sissy crossdresser or transgender woman, you can either politely and privately ask them--or you can not worry about it.

scenes & play

Negotiation

Good negotiation gives you and your partner the opportunity to have a better experience by clarifying consent, limits, and safewords. Fully-informed consent can't really be given or solicited if not everyone involved knows what's going on. It all starts with pre-scene negotiation; continues with ongoing, in-scene negotiation; and comes around to post-scene feedback. You and your partner should be communicating with and listening to each other continuously.

In her book, *Dom's Guide to Submissive Training*, Elizabeth Cramer explains why communication is so important in building a Dominant/submissive (D/s) relationship. Her thoughts apply equally well to age play interactions, whether they are D/s arrangements or not.

Because there is no standard way for people to come into BDSM and everyone has their own ideas about everything from the definition of words to the ways submission is practiced, it is important you have a spoken, agreed-upon and clear understanding of what you both want and expect.[1]

The word *negotiation* has come to hold special meaning within the BDSM community, beyond that found in the dictionary. It means a pre-play talk, which may be light and quick or lengthy and in-depth, in which people discuss their limitations, desires, and expectations. Most people engage in some sort of relationship negotiation when they're dating. They ask if the other person wants kids, what their interests are, what their schedule is like, etc. to see if this is a good fit and if they're willing to make the required sacrifices in order to fit into a relationship with this person.

Negotiating a scene is the same sort of thing: you usually sit down together, in your adult headspace, and talk about what you're into to some degree (interests, fetishes, and kinks), what you have no desire to do (limitations), and what you want to happen in the scene (expectations). You might also ask about someone's experience and even formal training, especially if you're going to be engaging in some sort of play that requires special skills, like play piercing or suspension bondage.

I like to ask about experience even if we're just hanging out, because it helps me to form a connection with my playmate. I find that newer players may need more guidance and that more experienced players may have stronger expectations, though that isn't always the case. Sometimes newbies are very, very certain that all scenes go a certain way. Sometimes more experienced players have learned that things work best for them if they really allow their playmate to lead play--even if the playmate is the submissive party.

Negotiation is where all that self-exploration discussed earlier comes in handy. After all, you can't very well tell someone who you are and what you're about if you don't know, even if what you learned was that you're still exploring and figuring things out. After you've introduced yourself to your (potential) partner and been introduced to them, you can get more into clarifying consent and planning out play, assuming that you both want to.

On my first date with my current partner, I asked what his orientation was. Baffled, he responded, "I'm...straight? You're bisexual, right?" I answered that I was a pansexual, masochistic, polyamorous, cisgender, switch, bottom age player who enjoyed a number of fetishes. I usually wouldn't open with that rather long list, but we were on our way to have sex, so it seemed to be a pressing detail. I also coaxed a few more answers out of him and learned that he was a heterosexual, monogamous, cisgender service top who enjoyed power exchange, was mildly sadistic, and never, ever subbed, though he sometimes liked to bottom for pain play. We weren't a perfect match, but we were able to find a way to fit together and had a lovely time. Since then both of our sexualities have continued to develop and grow together.

I mention this for two reasons: First, a lot of people don't have the vocabulary to communicate their interests, limits, sexual preferences, and gender in a meaningful way. Because of this, negotiation may involve some education, but you can usually get an answer out of them if you take the time to draw them out--and they're amenable to it. Second, just because you aren't a perfect fit doesn't mean that you can't find some common ground and have an amazing time.

Don't let anyone tell you that having flat out negotiations has to be awkward in any way. Yes, you may like surprises, but knowing that you are respecting your partner's limitations doesn't preclude that. Good communication really will give you a better experience, I promise. If you doubt that, I would ask you to think about why.

A big part of communication is paying attention to and responding to your partner's cues. It helps to have a shared vocabulary, trust, and the ability to ask and answer questions while still being respectful of someone's desire for privacy. This might sound a little tricky, but it can be learned with a little effort. I daresay that it's an innate ability for many people. If you can tell that your questions or revelations are making someone uncomfortable, you can always try to talk about it, take a break, or simply wish them well and then walk away. Not everyone is a good fit for everyone else. You can always try again later or with someone else.

If someone continuously asks questions that make you uncomfortable, tries to negotiate play that you've already declined, etc., then that person isn't really communicating or negotiating with you: they're trying to gaslight you, bully you, or wear you down. Make tracks.

If you're neurodivergent or have some social issues, you might want to inform your partner. Then they can either do some research on their own or you can direct them to media that you've found to be helpful in the past.

Consent, Limits, & Safewords

Consent should be clearly stated and enthusiastic. If someone seems reluctant or conflicted about playing with you, let them off the hook by suggesting that you do something else or asking to reschedule. Things might work out okay, but you don't want to be the type of person who goes around using shaky consent as a premise to pressure people into doing things that they don't really want to do. So pay attention to how your potential partner is communicating with you as well as the actual words that they're saying.

When giving consent, be clear. You may want to roleplay scenes that involve coercion or even rape fantasies, but you can do that later. During negotiation, do your best to leave no room for doubt that you want to do something.

Don't forget to define your desires as well as your limits, but be sure to define limits, whether hard or soft. (A "hard limit" is something that you have no interest in doing; a "soft limit" is something that you will only do under certain conditions, to please your partner, or grudgingly.) Everyone has sexual limitations and stipulations. If someone tells you that they have no limits, what they're really telling you is that they're a poor communicator.

However, if you're having trouble thinking of any relevant limitations, just negotiate the play that you're going to do, then stick to that. You won't always be able to think of every relevant limitation that you'll have and you may change your mind halfway through a scene. This is completely okay. If your partner is worth having, their desire to maintain a consenting, respectful relationship will outweigh any disappointment at hearing your safeword.

Consent should be continuous. Make it clear to your partner that you understand that either of you can withdraw consent at any time, for any reason, be it a physical, emotional, or practical concern, either with clear communication or a safeword. What is a safeword? It's a word that you use to let you partner know that you want to end play. It isn't specific to bottoms or Littles, it isn't specific to women, and it isn't specific to physical pain. Anyone can use a safeword for any reason at any time.

I encountered one of my favorite non-BDSM examples of a safeword in 2014 when I attended the Great Horror Campout in Sacramento. It was an overnight camping trip where attendees would run a horror-themed obstacle course. Performers would often get really close to attendees, even touching them directly or with props. There was even a van labeled "Free Candy" that was driven around by two big, burly men. If these guys spotted you, they would would jump out, grab you, and drive you around for 10 to 15 minutes with a black bag over your head before depositing you somewhere else, dazed and disoriented. Unsurprisingly, the Campout's organizers recognized that attendees needed a way to communicate a withdrawal of consent to the performers, just in case. They did this by informing everyone of a safeword, one that tickled me pink: "I want my mommy!"

Work out a safeword for yourself and your partner, whether you are topping or bottoming. Practice using it before your scene. If you're a top, you may want to check in with your bottom by periodically asking them, "Do you remember your safeword?" just to remind them that they can use it whenever they like. Discuss what you both expect to happen if you use your safeword. Does it mean that you need to check in and receive verbal reassurance? Does it mean that all play should cease immediately? Does it mean that you need to speak out of role?

Popular safewords include "mercy" and "red". It is generally understood within the BDSM community that using either of those words will bring play to an immediate stop. In fact, if you're in a public dungeon and someone yells either of those words and play does *not* stop, a dungeon monitor will probably stop your scene for you just to make sure that everything is consensual.

The color safeword system is modeled on traffic lights, where "red" indicates that play should stop, "yellow" indicates that play should proceed with caution, and "green" affirms that everything is fine. Some players find graded safewords like these to be quite helpful, especially if you're trying to get to know a new partner. After all, a mistake doesn't have to end play. Sometimes you can just adjust and keep going. Grading enthusiasm on a scale from one to five (or ten) can work well, too. I personally find it to be more helpful in scene than during pre-scene negotiation.

I really like safewords. I think they're an opportunity to have some fun and they can be a really hot negotiation tool. My favorite pornographic representation of safewords comes from A. N. Roquelaure's *The Claiming of Sleeping Beauty*. If such fantastical erotica can work clear-yet-coded communication into its story, you should do just fine working it into your scene.

> *"When I ask you will say, 'Only if it pleases you, my Prince,' and I shall know the answer is yes. Or, 'Not unless it should please you, my Prince,' and I shall know the answer is no. Do you understand me?"* [2]

I had a dream once, about which I couldn't wait to tell to my boy, Sam. In it, he, his girlfriend, and I were in a hotel room, ready to have sex. I was being very dominant with both of them and had her lie down on the bed with her legs spread. I positioned him over her and was ready to penetrate her with his cock when I realized that we didn't have a condom and they weren't fluid bonded. Instead of awkwardly ending the scene and running downstairs to get condoms, which is what I would have done in real life, I asked him, "Did you do your homework?" He said that, yes, he had. I asked her the same question and she also said that she had. Then I pushed his bare member into her.

Upon being told this story in the morning, they both made it clear that they would have used their safe word in that situation. However, we did take something of value away from my early morning sex dream: that's the phrase that I use now to solicit consent from my boy mid-scene without breaking character. I tend to be a very spontaneous Mommy and I haven't always gotten Sam's consent for everything that I want to do to him, so this works out very well for us. If he tells me that he hasn't done his homework, we don't do whatever crazy thing I've suddenly taken it into my mind to do. Instead he may get a spanking or maybe I'll tell him that he really should go do it, oh, after I have just one more orgasm. It's a safeword that I can solicit during a scene, though he can also randomly tell me that he just remembered that he has to do his homework. The point is, it works and it's *hot*. Other age play-style safewords that you might find titillating include, "You're not my *real* dad!" and, "I'll tell on you!"

Be aware of your situation and adjust safewords accordingly. If someone has a ball gag in their mouth, they probably can't use a safeword very effectively. Instead, they can start humming "Twinkle, Twinkle, Little Star" or even just humming tunelessly. Safe actions, that is non-verbal age play safewords, include dropping a stuffed animal or ball that you're holding, spitting out a pacifier, sucking your thumb, and looking into your partner's eyes while biting your lip, though this last one can be a bit subtle.

Sometimes you'll find yourself in negotiations with someone--or even fully in a scene--and you want to end it without being rude. It's completely okay to tell a little white lie or to make an excuse. If you're more of a straight shooter, I usually go with, "You know, I just don't think we're a good match." However you choose to end that particular conversation, don't feel bad about it. The only reason to do any of this stuff is that you want to. There is no obligation whatsoever.

Feedback

After a scene, you and your partner might want to give each other some feedback on how play went. This feedback may or may not be distinct from aftercare. You may be the type of person who prefers leisurely pillow talk while still clasped in your partner's arms or you might be more into a formal discussion over tea. Maybe it's just a practical discussion that takes place the next day as you're tidying up the kitchen together. I usually prefer to give feedback in the moment, during play. It feels more natural and playful and the payoff is immediate. It also helps to practice actually, say, taping a diaper on correctly rather than just talking about it and trying to make adjustments later on. Of course, you can always have play sessions that are centered on troubleshooting as well.

Regardless of the setting in which you give your partner feedback, try to be positive. Sometimes you just can't, but a good, understanding, sympathetic attitude can help to remind an embarrassed or even upset partner that you desire and respect them even as you're, well, complaining. (Of course not all feedback is negative, but the parts that you need to work to put a positive spin on usually are.) Express your desires productively, without being whiny or dehumanizing your partner. You two--or three or however many--are trying to create a positive experience and the best way to do that is with underlying respect and compassion. Be grateful that you have a partner to experience this stuff with and be open to compromising, adjusting, and learning. End on a genuinely good note with a sincere, meaningful compliment if at all possible.

Littles as Tops

Littles can make amazing tops. Remember your time on the playground? Kids can be *mean* and age players have the life experience to back up that curiously cruel attitude. Beyond simple teasing and spoiled behavior, Littles can order their Bigs or other playmates to do all sorts of things. I'm a big fan of Be My Slave for a Week, especially in exchange for sexual favors. I've also discovered that I really enjoy receiving oral sex while I play video games. It's oddly empowering.

In case you've forgotten those years on the playground or just managed to escape the notice of the meaner kids, here are some suggestions for Little bullies:

- Dangling spit: Hold your partner down and pretend that you're about to spit on them, only to suck it in at the last second. (Or not.)
- Indian burns: Grasp the skin on the forearm with both hands, then twist in opposite directions.
- Keep away, aka monkey in the middle: Recommended for three people or more; take something precious to one partner and play catch over their head.
- Pantsing: Yank down your partner's pants without warning! Try to do it *without* getting the underwear for extra points.
- Swirlies: Push your partner's head into a toilet and flush it, causing their hair to swirl around in the water.
- Tickling: Tickle your partner, maybe even until they pee!
- Wedgies: Grasp your partner's underwear firmly in your hand and yank it up between the buttocks. You can go for a frontal wedgie as well.
- Wet willies: Lick or suck on your finger to wet it with spit, then stick it in your partner's ear. For a green willie, use a booger instead of spit.

As with everything in this book, engage in the above only at your own risk and after acquiring informed consent via negotiation!

The first time I went to our local Littles Munch at Wicked Grounds, a San Francisco-based kinky coffee shop that boasts a special Littles menu, I had the good fortune to see a Little top in action. I don't know that she would have called herself that, but she totally was! The whole munch I don't think she moved more than to reach for a crayon, yet her Daddy (slave) brought her hot chocolate, cupcakes, and other treats. He fetched coloring books, tied her shoes, and cleared away dishes. He didn't do a single one of these things on his own, either. Instead, he waited for his princess to issue a command. I'd never seen such a devoted sub!

Turning Mommy or Daddy into a doll is a great way to kick off an impromptu tea party. Trust me: they're only pretending that they hate that sparkly tiara and pink feather boa. If the Little has earned their knot-tying badge, maybe Mommy or Daddy can even be tied to the chair! After all, parents can be kinda sneaky and don't always stay where you put them.

Solo & Long Distance

My guess is that most people who engage in solo age play would rather be age playing with a partner instead. Yet there are those of us who, even if we have the option of playing with others, choose to spend some quality time exclusively with our Little, perhaps decompressing from the community or just indulging in regression that is wholly focused on the self. Others don't feel social time to be all that essential to their Little incarnations. Or perhaps age play feels pretty purely sexual and sharing it would be like masturbating in a group. (Which is something I'm personally fond of, but I get that it isn't for everybody!) No matter the reason, there's certainly a large contingent of solo age players, who may never in their lives age play in front of another person.

Solo age play can be incredibly fulfilling. After my divorce, I was afraid that I would never be able to age play again. The idea of solo age play was terrifying. I had long gotten over the idea that being an adult choosing to wear a diaper was in any way weird, but diapering *myself* still felt...odd. But I was jonesing hard for some regression and diaper time, so I started experimenting and figured out what worked for me--and what didn't, but might still be a good idea for others.

I found myself cycling through regular life until I would become overwhelmed with desire to age play. But I wouldn't have anything planned or prepared, so I'd have an unsatisfactory masturbation session that would tide me over for a while and keep pushing through until the next time.

The problem was that I wasn't making time for a fulfilling age play experience. I started thinking of it as necessary, unnegotiable Me Time. Rather than a day at the spa, I would spend a day at the nursery. I began scheduling immersive age play experiences every two weeks. I would get little age play bumps in between by watching porn, reading stories, listening to MP3s, etc., but my bi-monthly sessions were what sustained my Little self.

An an exercise, try to think of solo age play as being in a long distance relationship with yourself. This was easy for me because I'm a switch, but even if you aren't, you may still want to try to develop an imaginary caretaker persona so that you can plan out your Little time specifically as a Big. It allowed me to feel cared for and answerable to someone. It might work for you, too!

Here's a sample schedule that I use when I engage in some solo school girl age play:

School Schedule

Wake Up I like to set an alarm clock for my schoolgirl days, which is something that I do only rarely in my everyday life. I don't set the alarm for particularly early because I do like to sleep in. If I wake up before my alarm, that means that I have time to masturbate. If my alarm goes off before I climax, I like to pretend that it means that

Mommy walked in on me, which usually leads me to finish up pretty quickly!

Ablution I take a bubble bath, comb my hair, and brush my teeth, using items conducive to age play, like a princess toothbrush. My hair is styled in braided pigtails with bows.

Dress The night before, I lay out my school uniform, a green plaid number purchased from frenchtoast.com. I wear cute, juvenile earrings and minimal other jewelry, maybe a locket or charm bracelet.

Breakfast I usually indulge in sugar cereal, hot chocolate, or toaster pastries. Or I might make an enormous American breakfast with bacon, sausage, eggs, and Mickey Mouse pancakes with M&M's.

Before School I'll watch the cartoons from my childhood until First Bell, which I usually set for 10:30 am. I set my phone's alarm to a ringing bell sound to go off throughout the day to mimic a school's bell system.

Lecture Years ago I found a wooden, adult-size school desk for sale at a thrift store. I keep it stocked with notebooks, textbooks, binder, pens, pencils, etc. A simple binder is a more compact solution if you can't have a fully stocked desk. I've also mounted a blackboard on the wall beside my desk. I usually write a message on it, like, "Welcome, class!" and the date. The day starts with the original version of the Pledge of Allegiance. Then I watch lectures from Kahn Academy, Crash Course, or other free, online educational services as I take notes. This is usually a very productive time. I think that a lot of adults would benefit from some sort of self-imposed study regimen.

Physical Education When I was in Japan in 2014, the first thing I picked up were some fetish gym bloomers. These coupled with a little white t-shirt, knee socks, and Converse sneakers constitute my gym uniform. The bloomers are also equipped with a zipper at the crotch. I cannot stress enough the usefulness of this feature. I even wear it with a diaper, where the zipper makes it even more fun to check the diaper's wetness indicators.

Test and Essay I spend some time taking a few tests that I've downloaded and printed, and writing an essay. These will be left on my nightstand so that I can grade them as a Big later. At this point, I'll retrieve my old tests from my binder and see how I did. A good score usually means some sort of predetermined reward, like ice cream after dinner. A bad score can mean clothespins on my nipples. (I don't often do light age play. It's all pretty dark down here.)

Lunch This is, naturally, out of my *Lost in Space* lunch box, packed the night before. I might try to have this in public. I usually tone down my attire before going out. I'm very shy and don't want to offend anyone or invite awkward questions. I prefer to get lost in my own little age play world.

Recess This is usually time for some sort of sexual game or indulging in a fantasy scenario that I've concocted. This is usually the climactic point in my scene and varies according to what I'm in the mood for.

Study Hall It's nice to have some time to just read fiction, relax, and enjoy being in a school uniform. If I'm feeling masochistic, I'll sit in my desk or even kneel on rice, but I usually get a little lax at this point and just curl up on my bed with some milk and cookies.

School's Out My schoolgirl persona lives in a world of perpetual Fridays. I'll take a walk around my apartment's block so that I can "come home" (and get out of the house a bit) and throw my backpack in the corner, toss my clothes all over my room, and get into a more babyish outfit, like feetie jammies or a onesie. "Homework" usually consists of getting actual work done, like updating my websites and blogs or organizing my mailing lists.

Tykables (née Snuggies) diapers include a cute bedtime checklist on their overnight diapers' packaging. It lists activities such as checking for monsters and plugging in your phone. It's absolutely precious!

You might want to consider creating what I call a *Thief of Always* schedule. In Clive Barker's *The Thief of Always*, each day was divided up into the highlights of a year: the day started with New Year at midnight, progressed through spring. By noon it was summer, dusk was Halloween, and evening was Christmas. You can set up your day to hit those same high points or perhaps to allow you to "grow up" or regress over the course of a day.

Another option is to create a list of rules to abide by for a set period of time. I have a set of these types of rules for my boy when we go to Disneyland. I enforce them while he abides by them, but he could certainly use them for a solo adventure.

Disneyland Rules

- Age-appropriate media only, including smart phone games, reading material, and social media.
- Always wear Mickey Mouse ears when in public.
- Bedtime is 10:30 pm.
- Bubble baths only, no showers or regular baths.
- Must color when waiting in restaurants.
- Must sleep with special stuffie.
- Must suck thumb on all dark rides.
- Must wet diaper on scary rides.

- No big boy underwear!
- Sippy cups only.

Even if you can't set aside an entire day, you can still make plans to spend an evening coloring, watching a movie, wearing a diaper, or reading your favorite children's book. If you can't even do that, at least spend fifteen minutes window shopping on your favorite age play websites, check out some age players on Twitter, or watch some YouTube videos. The Littles community has formed quite a presence on YouTube in recent years and there are lots of fun videos of people just hanging out and being Little!

You can also try not thinking of age play as selfish or wasted time. After all, when did you stop being important? Use age play to focus on self improvement. Read that book that may not benefit you in a practical way, but will help make you a more rounded, more interesting person. Learn a new skill while in Little mode. I like to indulge in age play when I have a tiresome chore to do. Doing the laundry because I need clean clothes is boring, but doing it as a chore to earn stars toward a reward is quite fun!

Long distance relationships are seemingly quite common in the age play community. It's hard to find someone to play with in person, after all. I've already mentioned thinking of solo age play as being in a long distance relationship with yourself. Most of what I've described above can be arranged long distance by a Big in terms of chores, tasks, webcam dates, and structure. Some other things that you and your Big (or you alone) might want to do to promote Little space include:

- Ask for a bedtime diaper. Whenever my boy is out of town, I like for him to come home to find a nice, thick overnight diaper waiting on his bed, sprinkled with baby powder, and bearing a lipstick print in my signature Rapture Rose color right over the crotch. I've also sent diapers like this one as care packages to clients so that they can feel as though I'm putting them in their bedtime diapers at night.

- Fill in a baby book. Search online or even in local thrift shops to find a cute baby book and fill it out for your Little self.

- Finish a coloring book. Choose something that requires you to color a page in your coloring book. The catalyst can be every time you miss your Big, every time you wet a diaper, every evening, etc. Then, when your coloring book is full, write a sweet message on the title page, give it a kiss, and send it off to your Big.

- Make a care package. Put together a care package for your Big. You can add things grown ups like, like coffee, scented candles, and, I dunno, a newspaper? Send them something cute that you've made, too, like some macaroni art or popcorn seasoning mix. Because I'm spoiled, I like to include a list of presents that a Big might send back to me!

- Pick out a bedtime story for your Big to read over the phone or on webcam.

- Play games online. Maybe your Mommy will teach you how to play chess over Skype. Maybe you both really enjoy a certain game on your smart phones.

- Record an MP3 of yourself saying, "I love you," or singing a nursery rhyme and send it to your Big.

- Set a special ringtone for your Big's text messages and calls, such as "My Heart Belongs to Daddy" or "Girl, You'll Be A Woman Soon".

- Start a wishlist and star point system. Make a wishlist on Amazon or other wishlist system and decide how many stars must be earned for each item. Keep track of how many stars have been earned on a physical, online, or smart phone star chart.

Scene Elements

In my experience, scenes work better when you take the time to set the mood. You can't always have a perfect environment and some people will never experience one, but even just cleaning up your room before you get started can help a lot. Try to think of things that you can do to all five of your senses to trigger regression.

Sight Tidy up the room that you're going to be Little in. Cover surfaces in cute, printed bedsheets, lay out fuzzy blankets, and arrange your toys, diapers, bottles, etc. nicely.

Smell Try to find some nursery (i.e. baby powder) scent and dab it on a few cotton balls, then place them around the room. You can also find candles and room sprays in a baby powder scent. Or perhaps you prefer the smell of chocolate, cinnamon buns, vanilla, or other sweet things.

Sound Put on some cute music. YouTube has plenty of free kids music compilations. My mentor, Natasha Strange, also showed me a lullaby application for your smart phone that will loop for a set period of time or even indefinitely. I really enjoy it as an innocuous background sound.

Taste I strongly prefer rubber nipples to silicone on my pacifiers and bottles. For me, the taste is a trigger for regression. You may also want to have a piece of a candy that you associate strongly with your childhood. My favorites are Werther's Original Hard Candies.

Touch Most age players will find many easily implementable touch triggers: the soft plastic of a diaper, a smooth and shiny rattle, a downy baby blanket, a cuddly stuffed animal. Enjoy touching the soft, clean items that you associate with being Little.

When planning out your scene, try to include a climax. Otherwise play will feel, well, anticlimactic. This climax can be sexual or it can be one of excitement. Diaper changes, expelling enemas, getting a new toy or outfit, or being spanked all serve as great climaxes. The scene can continue or not after the climax. I generally like to float down for a while after the climactic moment. If your climactic element is sexual, remember that your partner may be less interested or even completely disinterested in continuing a scene after orgasm has been achieved. Your mileage may, of course, vary.

The last scene element that I want to discuss is aftercare, which is the BDSM term for post-scene care that is emotional as well as physical. The purpose of aftercare is to recover and take care of your needs and those of your partner after an intense BDSM play or sex session. If your age play is relatively indulgent or relaxing, you might not see the point of aftercare, but even in these gentler situations, I still like to employ it for two reasons: 1. It helps to usher you back into the real world and your adult responsibilities. 2. A special ritual or routine for ending play and initiating aftercare can make the culmination of play more satisfying. Instead of being sad that play is over, you can still look forward to your aftercare.

When ending an age play scene, I like to do something adult like have a cup of tea, change into adult clothes, or sit down with a beer to discuss our play session. Even something as simple as hugging your partner and saying thank you can be effective. Cuddling is a pretty popular aftercare method, though, personally, it always makes me feel more Little than Big.

You can also negotiate aftercare *after* you play instead of before-hand. You don't always know what you're going to want to do upon completing a scene. And be sure to check in with your partner, so that they can get whatever they might need from you. Bigs, tops, and doms need aftercare, too!

On the other hand, age play itself can serve as aftercare, in particular loving, caring age play following an intense BDSM session. For example, a nice, thick diaper with baby powder can soothe a spanked bottom, especially with a little arnica oil or vitamin E rubbed into the skin. Top it off with a cute onesie, stuffed animal, warm blanket, and lots of cuddles from your Big and you have a truly decadent aftercare session.

Age Play Activities

Below you'll find a list of vanilla, kinky, sexual, and innocent activities for Littles. Hopefully this will help you out if you're looking for something to do during age play beyond just feeling Little or if you find that you've fallen into a rut.

Baking Making sweets is only half the fun. You can also decorate them! If your Big isn't around to supervise you, you can ask for a Little-friendly Easy-Bake oven.

Bathtime Jazz up bathtime with bubble bath, blown bubbles, water coloring tablets, toys, water guns, and more. I always like to bring my I Rub My Duckie vibrating rubber ducky. You may want to suggest that your Big bring a cute scrubbing mitt to make suds and a plastic cup to rinse them away. Smaller Littles may be able to fit a hooded character towel, too!

Battles One of the few ways I get to connect with my husband's Little side is by inviting him to mock battles. Even just handing him a tube of gift wrap can get him there. You've never seen someone look so adorable as they're bludgeoning you with a pillow or holding you down and administering a coup de grâce with a boffer sword. One of our regular household expenses are new darts for our NERF guns.

Battles crossover with crafting when I decide to play armorer. When I want to make something for my Daddy, I don't color a picture or bake cookies. I construct a crossbow out of pencils or use rolled paper to make a rubber band gun.

There's also room for BDSM within a play battle. My boy has his own foam sword and shield, both of which make handy spanking tools. I'm particularly fond of recreating a scene of "being bladed" from *The Sword in the Stone*, where I have him lie across my oversized stuffed dog and spank him with the flat of the blade.

Being Dressed Very few things make me feel more helpless than having someone else select my clothes and dress me like a doll. While I usually prefer diapers when I'm being Little, having my panties pulled up can also make me feel very Little. Having my shoes tied is another trigger for regression, but not necessarily vulnerability. I particularly enjoy untying my shoes, then forcing my boy to get down on his knees to fix it. It's also fun to rest a sippy cup on my Daddy's head when he does it. Sometimes I like to remind them who's in charge. (It's me.)

Blanket Forts Make a blanket fort for your Big. I prefer to restrict access to my very exclusive forts, possibly with a "No Boys Allowed" sign. Anyone trying to gain entry may have to prove their girl-ness by taking a special oath or showing their panties. "No Bigs Allowed" is another good fort rule, though it can be bent under special circumstances. For instance, if my Daddy wants in, he's going to have to do something for me, and it isn't going to involve pants. If he doesn't show an appropriate level of interest in gaining access to my awesome fort, he may soon find that he's misplaced his keys, wallet, laptop, or phone--or all four.

Board Games *Candyland* seems to be a favorite among age players, due to the simple rules and colorful, charming design. I have a limited edition in a tin box. The game can be sexualized with different colors drawn corresponding to different sexual acts. Another simplistic favorite is *Chutes and Ladders*.

Cardboard & Paper In the age of online shopping, many of us find ourselves with a surplus of cardboard around, which can be used to make models, dioramas, and even forts and castles. Cardboard weapons, armor, and costumes are fun, too. As for paper crafts, plain old paper airplanes and dolls are classics, along with origami. Perhaps you could use that cardboard to make a house for your DIY paperdolls. Wouldn't that be a feat sure to impress a Big?

Cartoons [adult swim] debuted in 2001, MTV aired a number of cartoons in the 1990s, and the good old Simpsons have been around since *The Tracey Ullman Show* shorts started in 1987. There are a lot of cartoons designed to appeal to adults and I can't even get started on all the cartoons aimed at chronological children. What I'm particularly excited about, at least in this context, are animated shows and movies that appeal to both adults and children, cartoons that a Little's mature mind can get lost in while still feeling that juvenile spark.

Cartoon Network has come out with a number of shows that fit into this category. *Steven Universe*, *The Amazing World of Gumball*, *Adventure Time*, *Chowder*, *Dexter's Laboratory*, and *Courage the Cowardly Dog* are some of my personal favorites. Other networks have made contributions as well. Nickelodeon's *Spongebob Squarepants* and *Fairly OddParents* stand out. Don't forget classics like *Rugrats*, *Animaniacs*, and *Rocko's Modern Life*. Lauren Faust's *My Little Pony: Friendship is Magic* and Alex Hirsch's *Gravity Falls* deserve a mention as well.

As an aside, comic books based on cartoons make, in my opinion, some of the best comic books for age players. They're the perfect mixture of interesting and innocent. I especially recommend *The Simpsons* comics and the graphic version of *The Last Unicorn*.

If your Little tends to be quieter and calmer, my recommendations would include *The Triplets of Bellville*, *The Secret of Kells*, *The Thief and the Cobbler Recobbled*, *Coraline*, and anything by Studio Ghibli. Winsor McCay's 1914 short *Gertie the Dinosaur* is great for age play scenes set in the early 1900s. And then there's Pixar! Even as lauded as it is, I've always felt that Pixar doesn't get enough respect in age play circles, at least not outside of *Frozen*.

I could talk about cartoons for ages and I often watch them for my own enjoyment as an adult, and with my chronological children. The difference is, whenever I'm watching cartoons in as a Little, I focus entirely on the cartoon. I make a point of not multitasking *at all*. No cooking, writing, making lists, or cleaning--just cartoons. I don't even color. I just let go and sink down into the animated world and feel my Little glow. Perhaps you also have a passion that spans all of your personae, that your Little self enjoys in a way unique from the way your Big self enjoys it.

Coloring & Painting Yes, you can just use a coloring book, but coloring can go beyond the page. Color on yourself, with washable markers, body paint, or even liquid latex! Sidewalk chalk is not only fun, but can look really cool in front of your house or parking space. Fingerpaints can be as sexy as they are messy. If you're going for that authentic elementary school vibe, get yourself some watercolors. They work on paper or as body paint!

Adult coloring has become a "thing" recently. I like to use this as a catalyst to advocate for something that has annoyed me for ages in the age play community: *neat coloring by Littles*. Differentiate yourself from the hipsters and *get messy*. Don't color in the lines. Use oversized crayons and hold them in your fist. Get washable crayons and spread the art to your walls. If you want to give yourself more of a challenge, use your non-dominant hand and color while looking in a mirror. Hell, use your feet! Lose yourself in the experience by all means, but make it a challenge, and challenge your adult proclivity to be neat.

If you don't want to have a coloring book in the house, you can search for coloring pages on your favorite search engine's image search. Try specifically looking for large format, black and white images. You can also make your own coloring book this way, adding pictures to be colored to a binder folder and completed pages to plastic page protectors. And don't underestimate drawing your own pictures. This is my favorite way to go.

As a side note, coloring is one of those background activities for Littles events. Over the years I've learned just how antisocial coloring can be. Yes, you can have Littles sort of coloring together and there's nothing wrong with that if you do, but I like to suggest that munches and newer events don't have coloring corners and that newer Littles don't bring coloring things to their first events. It's easy to use coloring as an excuse to not socialize or even make eye contact. Playing a game or talking are much better ways to connect.

Crafts Doing a craft is a great way to get into the mood for age play: it requires planning, special shopping, and yields a physical reminder. Follow a craft blog or use a search engine to find craft details. To get you started, crafts that your Little might want to try include:

- Baby name bracelets
- Craft stick cabins and picture frames
- Crayon art
- Crocheting
- Friendship bracelets
- Jewelry made out of Froot Loops or dyed macaroni
- Mason jar snow globes
- Pacifier clips
- Playdough (make it at home and add glitter, cinnamon, and food dye!)
- Puppets
- Salt dough ornaments
- Shrinky Dinks
- Timeout glitter bottles

Dressing Up Wearing age play clothes is sort of dressing up in itself, but you can take it beyond that. Buy or make some fairy wings! Watch *Star Wars* while wearing your stormtrooper mask! Chances are you have something cute in the back of your closet that you don't wear as often as you want to. You may even want to take some pictures and show off your outfit on your Little's social media accounts.

Glow-in-the-Dark My husband's rarely-seen Little self really enjoys playing with glow-in-the-dark toys. They're often on sale at Target in the one to three dollar section. They have plain bracelets, but they also have glow-in-the-dark toys, like swords and fairy wands. Whenever we go on an age play vacation, we take a pack of glow-in-the-dark stars to stick around the hotel room and make it feel more magical. As a tip, glow-in-the-dark bracelets and glow sticks will last longer if you place them in the freezer when you're done with them. Sometimes you can get two or three uses out of them.

Hairstyling & Brushing Hairbrushing is, in my opinion, a very underrated age play act. It's incredibly intimate and something that rarely happens to adults. After I've had a bath, my Daddy will usually brush my hair, which is quite a task with my thick curls that reach nearly to my waist when straightened. I also really enjoy braiding, at least for girl-girl age play sessions when I won't also have to teach the person to braid and risk getting my locks hopelessly tangled.

Medical Play Does your Little like to play doctor? Are you curious about what's in the other adult kids' pants? You can always ask your Big to give you a medical exam, possibly including an enema, rectal temperature taking, and even nasty medicine, but you can also procure a play doctor's kit and give them one.

I don't have the patience to actually do it, but I've always thought it would be fun to put an arm or leg in a cast before an age play party. Then I would show up with a bunch of markers and stickers so that the other Littles could help me decorate!

What we *have* done at a local, Little Scouts age play party was to set up a Stuffie Hospital where Littles could bring their stuffed animals and other toys to be examined and repaired. We had a medical table stocked with various metal medical instruments, bandages, etc. Once your stuffie had been examined, you would also get a certificate verifying their health, to add to your medical records. It was a lot of fun and the Littles got really creative with their stuffies' ailments and injuries.

Outings When playing in public, keep discretion in mind. The world is not your nursery or dungeon or whatever. Be respectful of public places. Do not push your kink into others' faces. That said, Littles can have an amazing time in public, like at the annual LittleSpace Disneyland trip. Not that you have to go out with a group. Solo outings to parks, attractions, and museums can be a lot of fun, too. Even just a trip to the movies can be most enjoyable. Just be sure that you're keeping a low profile and being polite.

Pet Play You can be a cute little pet yourself or you can get your

Big or other friends to engage in a little roleplay. My Daddy makes a wonderful pony and even has a saddle. Note that pet players--cat boys and girls, kittens, human puppies and ponies, etc.--are usually considered distinct from the furry community. Hence, being a pet player is distinct from being a babyfur.

The playful energy of the pet play community often merges really well with that of the Littles community. Crossover events often do really well, with human ponies being brought out to be petted and adored or other pets being corralled into a human petting zoo. The San Francisco Pride Parade has gone so far as to make a point of marching Littles adjacent to the human ponies et al. The Littles were even encouraged to bring treats like sliced cucumbers and Skittles.

Most pet play events, like bath time and playing with toys, are analogous to how Littles spend their time anyway. I even see some crossover in my toy kits, including an oversized pacifier that is actually a chew toy. Scooby-Doo! Cinnamon Graham Cracker Sticks make excellent treats for Littles and pets alike.

Reading It can be difficult to find children's books that will hold an adult's attention. I usually recommend books for young adults instead of actual baby books. On the other hand, if your Little has a short attention span, cute baby books work great! And don't forget about bathtime books, which are made out of plastic so that you can take them into the tub.

Science Projects You can choose to just have fun with your science project, or you can choose to really *learn* something. As with all things, be responsible and safe! Here are some ideas to get you started:

- Add Mentos mints to soda pop.
- Grow crystals from sugar.
- Grow some mold.
- Make a periscope.
- Make a pinhole camera.
- Sculpt a vinegar-and-baking-soda volcano.
- Take a spore print from a mushroom.

Shopping Sometimes shopping is a reward for Littles, other times it's a punishment--and you can't always tell which it's going to be until you're there. Sitting on a chair, holding Mommy's purse, and staring at the wall after having your phone taken away is probably not what most Littles realize is the reality of going lingerie shopping.

Shopping doesn't have to be a form of financial domination either. Just take a normal shopping trip, say to the grocery store. As a Big, I like to keep some cheap toy, maybe a Hot Wheels car or a little sticker book or something, tucked into my bag. Throughout the trip it can be used to motivate my Little to behave.

Then again, shopping trips can be all about financial domination. This may not seem like an area that easily blends with age play, but it does. Bigs can issue their Littles an allowance or set the terms of a strict budget. It can be reversed in a Little handing over their earnings to their Big because, well, Littles aren't allowed to have money!

Snack & Meal Time Breakout the plastic dishes and make yourself some Star Wars mac-n-cheese or some microwave dinosaur chicken nuggets. If you're interested in making yourself a bottle to go with that, you probably want to avoid actual baby formula, except as a punishment. It tastes awful. Go with strawberry, chocolate, or plain milk. If you want something that tastes like milk, but involves the ritual of making formula, get yourself some powdered milk, then warm it up. For additional verisimilitude, don't use the microwave. Instead, ask your Big to warm your milk in a bottle warmer or saucepan with water--and be sure that your Big tests it on their wrist to see if it's too hot.

Dolls, Stuffed Animals, & Action Figures Playing with dolls, stuffies, and action figures can be almost hypnotic. If you can get deep enough into Little space, or if you have a very strong imagination, you can completely lose yourself in a fantasy that you've created. If you need a little more stimulation and have time on your hands, you can always get into the game of restoring thrifted toys or crafting your own.

Swimming Besides the normal joy of playing in water and all the cool water toys, age playing in water can be very fulfilling. Flotation allows for play that might usually be difficult or impossible, like being carried or rocked by someone who may not be quite strong enough to do so on dry land.

Tea Parties Your tea party can be an elaborate real-world affair with invitations and guests--or it can be an even more elaborate imaginary affair with stuffie guests and "just pretend" tea. Tea parties can allow your Little to engage in a lot of other activities in order to prepare, if you want to go that route. Or it can just be a moment to feel fancy in a Little way. For Littles who aren't allowed caffeine, but still want tea at their tea parties, I like to serve white tea (boiled water) or crystal tea (boiled water with a spoonful of sugar stirred in). It's also less likely to stain, if that's a concern.

Tickling Tickling is another one of those activities that can be either a punishment or a reward. When negotiating tickle play, I like to clarify whether my partner is more interested in intense, tied-to-a-chair, pee-your-pants tickling or more sensual, trailing-fingertips, feather tickling. I always like to remind my partner that a safeword can be used for tickling, too. Keep in mind that certain areas of the skin, especially if they come in contact with deodorant, can be easily irritated and prolonged tickling can, indeed, lead to raw, exposed skin.

Dark Age Play

The definition of dark age play has always been a little muddled, but when people use the term, they usually mean one of four things: 1. Age play that is sexual. 2. Age play that includes classic BDSM or domestic discipline. 3. Age play that involves *especially heavy* classic BDSM. 4. Age play that is gothic in culture and aesthetic. The first two definitions seem to be the most common, though it certainly varies from social circle to social circle. Here, I'm going to use a melding of those two definitions.

While some practitioners of domestic discipline might cringe at my discussing it in relation to BDSM, I'm going to do so, because that's what it is. Others might find it surprising that there's any division at all over whether or not domestic discipline is a form of kink. Despite inaccurate definitions given by sex-negative writers or writers who specifically fetishize monogamous marriage, domestic discipline is indeed a version of D/s play: there is a dominant partner (the head of household) and a submissive partner (the taken in hand). It's a simple connection.

The domestic discipline community often uses its own charming vocabulary to describe play and has a lighter aesthetic, which I find to be very conducive to dark age play with innocent overtones. Certain incarnations of age play can fit even the most sententious definitions of domestic discipline.

Dark age play can manifest in the use of "pervertables" or innocent items that can be used in a sexual manner or vice versa. Pervertables can be purchased or crafted. For example, a pacifier gag can be made by simply securing a pacifier in place with some rope or duct tape, or it can be purchased from an etsy.com vendor.

Further examples of age play pervertables include:
- Baby bottles or sippy cups filled with more adult substances, possibly for forced intoxication scenes or the consumption of sexual fluids. (Be sure to slightly enlarge the holes of rubber nipples to accommodate adult mouths. I've even found it advisable to take a drill to the hard plastic holes of some sippy cup lids.)
- Being bound in a crawling position on the hands and knees, with the wrists connected to the thighs or knees. This position, of course, facilitates doggy style sex.
- Binding the pinkie and ring fingers together, and separately

binding together the middle and index fingers, reducing the Little's motor skills.

- Board, card, etc. games with sexual stakes, like strip Go Fish or replacing the dice in *Sorry!* with sex dice.
- Gagging the Little, perhaps with a small stuffed animal held in place with bondage tape, and reducing them to baby talk.
- Nipple clamp pacifier clips, possibly which have been attached to a cock ring.
- Locking plastic pants or diaper pins secured with zip ties.
- Mitts or booties secured with (locking) bondage cuffs. This not only forces the Little to wear babyish clothing, but restricts the use of the hands, allowing the Little only babyish motor skills.
- Pacifiers filled with sexual fluids, then placed in the freezer so that they can be slowly enjoyed.
- Plastic pants lined with minty pain relieving ointments. Be careful not to inflict a chemical burn and know what to do in case of accidents.
- Stuffed animals who have been upgraded with a strapon or vibrator.

Dark age play also often manifests as roleplay molestation, possibly with a veneer of consensual non-consent. Usually when I'm asked about this sort of thing, I'm not asked about what to do--people apparently have that bit figured out--but about how to make the experience feel more genuine. I feel that this issue is best dealt with on a personal basis, by people who know each other very well. However, there are little theatrical triggers that can help you to get started.

To trick your subconscious mind into feeling that twinge of realistic distress, you can try setting up your scene with greater verisimilitude. How does your fantasy go down? Let's say it happens right after lights out, as you're lying in bed. Go through your bedtime routine, say goodnight, and snuggle down in the darkness. Think about something else, anything. Think about elephants. Think about the smell of cinnamon. Think about a movie you just saw. Then react as you do in your fantasy, in keeping with your negotiations.

One of the things that I like to do in order to better simulate non-consent in a consensual situation is to have my husband, who doesn't drink, gargle with whiskey before our scene. The smell is powerful, threatening, and I strongly associate it with this type of play.

You can also carefully negotiate the use of a false safeword. Inverted color safewords, where "green" means stop and "red" means proceed work well, especially if you don't usually use color safewords and are protected from later confusion. *Negotiate clearly for every scene!*

In *The Age Play and Diaper Fetish Handbook* I talk about a lot of age play punishments, ranging from traditional spankings to more unusual sour dummies. (A sour dummy is made by injecting a pacifier with vinegar, lemon juice, or another sour solution before freezing it. The pacifier is then given as a sour-tasting punishment.)

Rather than repeat myself and talk more about age play punishments, I wanted to take this opportunity to talk about age play *as* punishment. Diapering and forced wetting and messing are pretty prolific punishments that I also go into in *The Age Play and Diaper Fetish Handbook*. However, age play punishments can be much more subtle.

For example, my boy hates being made to listen to childish music. I, on the other hand, don't mind it so much. I don't really like it, but I can tune it out. My boy is, naturally, a Little and usually an enthusiastic age player, but this one thing really throws him off and makes an excellent punishment, especially when we're in public or in the car. I can take him lingerie shopping and thoroughly mess with him by making him wear headphones and listen to kids' music while I paw my way through panties and bras.

Other media aimed at children make good punishments, too. In my experience, some forms of children's media lend themselves better to those of us with developed, adult minds than others. I love *Adven-*

ture Time, but have you ever tried to sit through an episode of *Blue's Clues*? It's torture. (If you like *Blues Clues*, well, I'm sorry. Very, *very* sorry.)

Embarrassing clothes are another way to use age play as a punishment, but you have to be a little more careful about offending someone. I suggest playing off innocent questions about an embarrassing item with a little white lie: "Oh, I lost a bet."

Some of my favorite items--besides diapers--are bibs and ruffled ankle socks. I also own a pair of bright pink sneakers with purple laces. No one seems to mind them, but they are pretty embarrassing. They were purchased after a pair of high heels became too uncomfortable, which added extra humiliation to the event. I couldn't cut it in big girl shoes, so I needed to buy and wear those embarrassing sneakers. Another embarrassing age play purchase was a purple t-shirt that I had made at a local printing store. It has a diaper on the front, over the words: "Livin' the dream." Luckily the staff didn't ask for an explanation!

Eating childish food or being served in a childish way is another great form of humiliation. My boy has a special water bottle that he drinks out of in public age play scenarios. If you don't want to or can't bring special age play dishes out with you to eat, just being fed by another person can be incredibly embarrassing, especially if it continues for the entire meal. And of course straight baby food or formula is a punishment in itself. Yuck!

Protocol & Rules

There are extensive opportunities for protocol either in age play relationships or in the creation and adherence to a personal code. Littles' lives are often defined by limitations, which probably has something to do with the stereotype that they are inherently sub-missive. I'm going to give examples of different rules and protocol systems that can be implemented for Littles, but these examples can also be implemented as household rules which Bigs adhere to as well. If your Big only wants to adhere to some of the rules set for you, there's no reason not to have two separate rule sets, one that's only for Littles and one that's for the whole household.

- Address Bigs by their honorific and surname, such as Mr. Bear or Mx. Leather. (When designing protocol that has to do with social interactions, remember that others may not want to participate in your protocol. Respect their wishes.)
- Address *your* Big only as Mommy, Daddy, etc.
- Bedtime is 10:00 pm.
- Earn at least three chore stars per day.
- Eat healthy food.

- Eat with cute plastic dishes and utensils.
- Greet your Big as they arrive home with a hug, kiss, and colored picture.
- Hold hands with your Big when crossing the street together.
- If you are with your Big, do not tie your own shoes or put on your own seatbelt. Ask your Big to do it.
- No drinking or smoking. (I also enjoy the rule, you may only drink alcohol if you are wearing a diaper.)
- Only sit in the backseat of the car.
- Only take bubble baths; no showers.
- Sleep with a stuffed animal.
- Suck on your pacifier whenever using your computer or watching TV alone or in suitable company.
- Wear diapers to bed.

If you find memorizing lists of rules to be tiresome, you can opt instead for a mantra that guides your behavior and mindset. It's easier to memorize, and it's more general meaning can be applied to all actions and thoughts.

Example Mantras

- "Daddy knows best."
- "Diapers are made to be used."
- "I can be as Little as I want to be."

- "My heart belongs to Mommy."
- "Sugar and spice and everything nice. That's what I'm made of."

I change rules according to my whim when I top and am admittedly absent minded about rules that I've set in the past. So instead of giving up or floundering all the time, I create rules for shorter periods of time. It's in better keeping with my lifestyle and I enjoy the glow of meeting daily or even hourly goals just as much as I enjoy living in a 24/7 dominant-submissive dynamic. A rule that I might come up with on the spot might sound something like, "You may only eat yellow and green foods today." Because these rules expire, I can make them especially difficult and peculiar if it amuses me.

If you have a particularly regimented relationship with your partner; be they Big, Little, or something else entirely; you might want to consider drafting a contract. Signing a contract, which is not legally binding, is common enough in the Leather community and among BDSM practitioners. There are various play contracts available online if you need some help in writing one.

My boy, Sam, is under contract indefinitely. In keeping with the age play tones of our relationship, he also has an adoption certificate marked with his registry number from slaveregister.com. I'm not able to adopt Sam legally. Laws vary from locality to locality, but in

California, an adoptee must be at least ten years younger than the guardian and they may not have had sex. Sam is, in fact, a month older than I am and we've had lots of sex. Instead, he offered me his power of attorney.

When writing a contract, I like to split it up into several parts:

- A disclaimer that states that the contract is not legally binding and is intended as a roleplay aid and communication tool. I also state that all changes must be agreed upon by both parties and that the issuance of a new contract necessitates the destruction of the old contract by burning. (Mostly because I like to burn things.)
- A list of my responsibilities to my partner. (I tend to joke around a lot as a dominant, so I include a sort of reverse safeword. If I say, "That is an order," then Sam knows that I'm being serious and I really do expect him to, say, drink from his baby bottle in the middle of the busy shopping mall.)
- A list of my partner's responsibilities to me.

CERTIFICATE of ADOPTION

THIS IS TO CERTIFY THAT _____

HAS ADOPTED _____

ON _____.

_____
Signature of Big

_____
Signature of Little

By signing this certificate, you agree to provide your adopted Little with affection, comfort, and care. In return, your Little will adore and obey you.

Take the time to design a cute, meaningful adoption certificate. It can be a surprise or something that you do with your Big!

- Clarification of safewords and limitations. Limitations may be specific, as in, no edge play without specific negotiation. They may also be general, as in, no play that may jeopardize my family situation.

- A pledge or vow written from the perspective of one or both (or all) involved parties which sets the tone of the relationship.

- Signatures, along with the date and, if any, the expiration date of the contract. Remember that contracts may only last a set period of time or regularly necessitate renewal.

Sam and I also have a section in our contract that defines different dynamics I might invoke to better fit our situation. We have a multi-dimensional relationship and my interests are varied. Hence, Sam may need to fill different roles. I refer to our basic dynamic as Sam being "in attendance". This is more or less how we are with one another at all times in everyday situations. When Sam is in attendance, he refers to me as "Mommy". He must obtain my permission to eat, drink anything other than water, use the restroom, and disagree with me. He is also expected to generally make my environment more pleasant by tidying up around me and bringing me water.

When we are in an adults-only environment conducive to age play, Sam is said to be "under care". When he is under care, I expect him to be dressed in a juvenile manner, wear diapers, and generally be more dependent upon me. Instead of asking to use the restroom as he would when in attendance, he would instead ask me to take him to the bathroom.

In professional or high fetish situations, I invoke "high protocol". At this time, Sam behaves more like an old guard Leather slave than a Little, though his attire usually makes it clear that he is, indeed, a Little. His prime objective is to serve me. Hence, he stands at attention at all times. He speaks only when spoken to, and then he does so sparingly.

I bring these variations up because I find that most people are overly ambitious when setting up their contracts. So, instead of limiting your ambition, I recommend that you're realistic about your abilities, but also include your fantasies. And remember that contracts can always be amended or altered later.

Sample Age Play Contract for Submissive Little & Dominant Big

Binding [name of Little] into the Care of the [name of Big]

This contract is in no way legally binding, and is meant only as an aid to a better understanding of the needs, duties, and responsibilities of the Little and Big. It is intended only to:

1. Enhance a roleplaying scenario between the involved parties.
2. Clearly state the full mutual consent of the undersigned.
3. Explain the responsibilities, duties, and limits of both the Little and Big.
4. Define the Little's safeword and its use. [While I make a point that Bigs may also safeword for any reason, I find that in events where a contract is drafted, my control over the Little is developed to the point that I determine all play and can simply stop or put the Little on time out if I want to. Hence, I don't feel the need to clarify my own safeword in a contract. Your mileage may vary.]
5. Foster a greater sense of communication between the

involved parties.

This contract may not be altered, except when both the Little and Big agree. If the contract is altered, the new contract shall be printed and signed, and the out-of-date contract must be destroyed.

Big's Responsibilities

The Big agrees to take charge of the Little, under the provisions determined in this contract. The Big agrees to care for the Little, to arrange for their safety and wellbeing, as long as they are under the Big's protection. The Big also accepts the commitment to treat the Little properly; to teach, punish, reward, and nurture.

The Big agrees to:
- Learn what excites the Little through exploration and communication and to try to incorporate these findings into the relationship.
- Make their desires and commands clear at all times.
- Only to accept other playmates and partners in consideration of their existing responsibilities toward the Little.
- Furnish the Little with a symbolic token of the relationship, to be worn by the Little at all times, except when to do so would be inappropriate.
- Discipline the Little only out of a desire to better them or to sensually enjoy them, and never out of anger or

frustration.

Little's Responsibilities

The Little agrees to:

- Obey the Big's rules to the best of their ability.
- Strive to overcome all inhibitions that limit their growth as a Little.
- Maintain honest and open communication.
- Inform the Big of desires and perceived needs, recognizing that the Big is the sole judge of how or if these shall be satisfied.
- Always address the Big as "Mommy" [or other pet name] unless otherwise instructed or when to do so would be inappropriate.
- Speak respectfully to the Big at all times, including times not spent in a scene.

The Little agrees to maintain their appearance and health, being clean, well-rested, and well-fed. When the Little dresses for the Big, clothes and hair are to be styled in the juvenile manner heretofore agreed upon.

The Little agrees to answer any and all questions asked by the Big freely, promptly, and to the best of their knowledge. They further agree to volunteer any information that the Big should know regarding the Little's physical or emotional state. The Big agrees to never use this information to harm the Little in any way.

In regard to treats and screen time, the Little renounces all rights to their own gratification except insofar as permitted by the Big. The Little may not seek any other dominant, Mistress, Master, owner, Big, et al. without the Big's clearly stated permission.

Limitations & Safeword

Nothing asked of the Little will demean them as a person and will in no way diminish their ability to fulfill professional or personal responsibilities or to reach their full potential. Nothing will be required that will in any way damage or harm the Little's relatives or friends, or interfere with the performance of their relationship duties.

The Little accepts the responsibility of using a safeword, "red," when necessary, for fear of jeopardizing anyone's physical, mental, emotional, financial, or any other safety. Use of the safeword will result in an immediate cessation of the worrisome activity.

The Big accepts the responsibility of complying with the Little's use of their safeword. The Big agrees never to punish the submissive for implementing this safeguard, but to encourage its use where appropriate. The Big also agrees to abide by any limitations held by the Little, including, but not limited to:

- No scat play.
- No vomit play.
- Edge play only with specific negotiation.

Should either party find that their aspirations are not being well served by this agreement, find this commitment to be too burdensome, or for any other reason wish to cancel this contract, verbal notification is sufficient for doing so, in keeping with the consensual nature of the agreement. Cancellation will result in a cessation of the control stated and implied within this agreement, not of friendship.

Big's Promise

I promise to protect, nurture, and love my Little to the best of my ability. I will do everything that I can to provide the type of care that will benefit them, even if that means that I must be strict and severe. My Little's fulfillment shall be my highest priority. I accept them as a child born of my heart and vow to hold them close now and until the cessation of this agreement.

Signatures

Big: I hereby accept responsibility for my Little under these terms stated above on this the _____ day of _____ in the year 20__. By the affixation of my signature, I promise to be dutiful and to fulfill the sweet and playful nature of my Little to the best of my abilities. I have read and fully understand this contract in its entirety.

Little: I hereby acknowledge that I belong to my Big under these terms stated above on this the _____ day of _____ in the year 20__. By the affixation of my signature, I promise to be dutiful and to fulfill the loving and caring nature of my Big to the best of my abilities. I have read and fully understand this contract in its entirety.

Age Play Collaring Collaring is a commitment ceremony held for partners in a BDSM relationship to formalize their connection. It's a bit like a wedding. As a Little, you may find yourself wanting to be ceremoniously (or not so ceremoniously) bound to your partner. Of course, like a wedding, you can more or less do whatever you want, but there are some semi-formal ceremonies which have formed within the age play community.

A classic collaring ceremony can always be held, with the collar be-ing one that reflects the aesthetics of the relationship. Retailers on etsy.com offer a number of collars dripping with lace, bows, bells, pacifiers, diaper pins, and other age play-evocative trinkets. There are collars engraved with "baby girl" and teddy bears. If you can't find something that you like, you can always craft one yourself or commission a custom job.

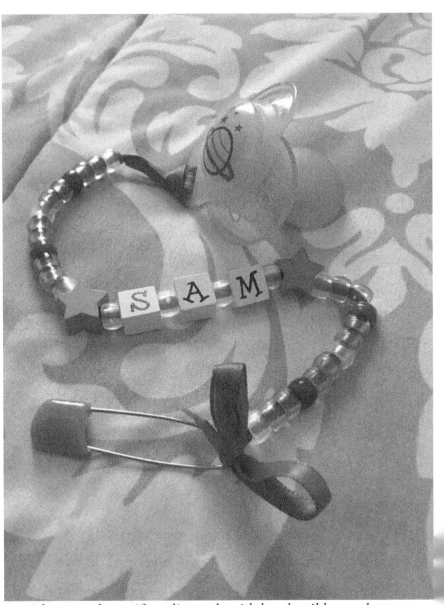

A homemade pacifier clip made with beads, ribbon, a button-pacifier holder, and a safety pin.

Your collaring ceremony could avoid an actual collar altogether. Al-ternatives include special pacifiers with clips either in plastic or sterling silver--or any other material you see fit and can afford. Baby items either plated in or made of sterling silver are numerous, ranging from hair clips to porringers. Sterling silver rattles and birth certificate holders look particularly fine when they are engraved with the Little's name.

Ceremonies common in the age play community include trips to Build-A-Bear Workshop to procure a special stuffie, vacations or day trips to Disney parks, and the crafting of custom pacifier clips. A trip to the jewelry store to select a special charm bracelet (and perhaps to begin the selection of charms for anniversaries or age play accomplishments), a locket, or perhaps to have an ID bracelet engraved would work well, too. I have yet to see an age play quinceañera or sweet 16, but I think it would be a marvelous idea!

Prepare for a Rainy Day

It's a bit of a downer, but it's important to be prepared for slumps in interest, losing your partner, or even being outed. Have a plan for what you'll do in each situation. Think about which friends might help you get through it and how you can bounce back.

Thinking about worst case scenarios can help you avoid a damaging knee-jerk reaction. You don't want to overreact or be completely crushed--and it can indeed be crushing to think that you've finally found someone who understands an unusual kink only to lose them.

Anyone who plays long enough will experience periods when they're simply not interested in play--and their partner will feel that way at times, too. It's just the way things are. Be prepared to have a talk with your partner about how you two might get back on track and start playing again, what might help charge your interest. Taking regular breaks from play can help keep you from feeling burnt out.

Roles

Given the diversity represented by an age, I always like to use roles and archetypes when negotiating play with others, as I feel that it better helps us to see how we might fit together.

Many roles will fit together clearly, such as a naughty schoolgirl and a strict teacher or a shy neighbor boy and the unscrupulous cougar next door. Others may require a little finesse, but I'm of the opinion that any two roles can be successfully fitted together. "The sadistic dentist and the hypochondriac girl scout" may not be a cliche yet, but once you say it out loud, it practically roleplays itself.

Roles that I've enjoyed are listed below, just to help you jumpstart ideas. I've included an elevator pitch for each to illustrate how you might describe your desired role to a potential playmate. Keep in mind that Littles can be tops! Roles are not inherently gendered!

Boarding School Bully I take advantage of the absence of parents and apathetic teachers to act like a tyrannical little queen. I may have a toadie to enforce my tiny edicts, but it's also likely that I'll just pound any challengers myself.

Clingy Preschooler I desperately don't want Mommy and Daddy to leave me alone with *strangers*. I bat my eyes and cuddle, wiggling around in my diaper and insisting that I'm still a baby and need to stay home and be bottle fed, changed, and cared for in every way.

Forcibly Regressed Girlfriend All my "big girl" privileges have been taken away. My dominant boyfriend has decided that what he really wants is for me to be completely at his mercy, ready to be "raised" and punished as he sees fit. I try to resist the spankings and restrictions, but I just can't. Maybe the thick diapers or frilly baby clothes are getting to me...

Ominous Little You've seen *The Omen*. You know where this is going, but I'll say it anyway: I'm a little terror, a sullen kindergoth who manipulates her caretakers and is even more dangerous than she is cute.

Overprotective Older Sister My beautiful younger sister is starting to get attention. But I've always put her and her sexual purity up on a pedestal, even if I don't have those standards for myself. I go out of my way to infantilize her and neutralize everybody who tries to worm their way into her ruffled panties.

Sexually Aggressive Neighbor Kid A chronic masturbator, I get other neighborhood kids alone and cajole them into playing a game with me, a game that Mommy and Daddy might not want us playing. But anyone who goes along with my little game will get to feel really, really good. I promise, it's better than all the candy and video games in the world!

Social Outcast with Overactive Imagination I'm lost in my own little world, but that's okay. Sometimes I might say weird things or stomp off on my own little adventure, my teddy bear backpack stuffed with PB and J, a crayon-drawn treasure map clutched in my sticky fist.

Try coming up with a pitch or two for your Little self to describe what you're like and give others ideas for connecting with you. Write it down if you like, tweak it, say it out loud. Get a really good, strong idea of who your Little is so that you can present yourself to the world with confidence and intent.

Resources

The following resources have been organized in the way that I thought they might be most useful. Sometimes that meant organizing them according to type of media. Other times it meant organizing them according to function. I have used a variety of citation styles as well, valuing usability over uniformity.

I tried to include resources aimed *exclusively* at adults, though some, like mainstream clothing companies and television shows, are only aimed *mainly* at adults. Then there are resources, mostly online stores, which sometimes fail to choose between providing fetish items and items for chronological children. While I am aware of these companies and understand that they may have some great products, I chose not to include them. Our community is already subject to misconceptions over whether or not Littles are a form of pedophile. If you come across one of these companies that use images of or reference chronological children, I encourage you to shop elsewhere and to petition them to remove the inappropriate material. Our community is small and fragile. Let's keep it safe and respectable by insisting on good, strong boundaries.

I also have tried to include only resources which are up-to-date at the time of writing, I have had personal experience with, and are the top in their fields. In short, this list is meant to be useful, not exhaustive.

Parker at babesindiapers.com is compiling a master list of all mainstream media references of women in diapers, diaper-like garments, and age play situations. He's also soliciting aid from the community, so if you know of something not already posted or can provide the provenance for an uncited work, please do inform him!

Because the Littles community is burgeoning, most well-developed resources are aimed at or at least use the language of the ABDL generation. Don't let that put you off! Just because you don't identify as an adult baby doesn't mean that you can't benefit from their resources.

In listing documentary works, especially movies and television, I tried to mention any negative impact that appearing on the program had for the participants. I've been asked to do a number of these programs and have almost always said no. I've even turned Howard Stern down. The reason is that I prefer to appear in media that is not only *about* age players and diaper fetishists, but *by* us as well. Given the current state of things, this usually means that the media is also *for* us, as with the Big Little Podcast.

If you are going to appear on any show, even one controlled by Littles or other age players, be sure to know what you're getting yourself into. Check out the program's previous work. Is it sensitive? Have past participants experienced negative fallout as a direct result? Are Littles being displayed for shock value or to be mocked? If so, just walk away.

Remember that you can always say no to anything and even change your mind after having said yes--so long as you haven't signed a contract to the contrary. My favorite example of this is at the end of *A Weekend at Miss Martindale's* when an off-camera woman asks Miss Martindale to tell the camera something about her childhood. Miss Martindale chirps, "No." The documentary ends on the sound of her silvery laughter. [1]

was once approached by a production studio to appear in a pilot for a reality show about life as an adult actress who was also a wife and mother. It paid a *lot* of money. I immediately asked if they would blur my chronological children's faces and use only pseudonyms.

They refused to answer me--again and again and again. Finally I put my foot down and said that I could not communicate with them further unless they answered my question. They finally informed me that I would need to sign a release exposing my children's identities. That was a hard limit for our family, so I declined. They handled it less than gracefully, but that was about what I expected after their callousness towards my children and unprofessional question-dodging. Do not be afraid to walk away from a deal in favor of something infinitely more valuable.

The National Coalition for Sexual Freedom offers a full list of media tips on their website.[2] Before you give your interview, review it and practice, practice, practice. Write out what you might say and memorize key phrases. Practice speaking in front of the mirror and any friends who might agree to help you. Plan out your attire and, if you have control over it, the interview room. Go in as prepared as possible.

Books & Articles

Ageplay: from Diapers to Diplomas by Paul Rulof (Lulu, 2011) It is clear from reading his work that Rulof is an educator and community leader. His book is approachable and includes a lot of anecdotes about age play scenarios and dynamics.

The Age Play and Diaper Fetish Handbook by Penny Barber (Lulu, 2011) In my first book, I mostly give practical advice about how to actually do things, like give an enema or fold a cloth diaper. If you are especially into diapers, cloth or disposable, this book can help you setting up your scenes.

The Babies by Susan Sontag, photographed by Polly Borland (powerHouse Books, 2001) Sontag and Borland have both worked on a number of interesting projects. The pictures in *The Babies* are not glossy fetish photos. They're depictions of real, delicate human beings--mostly older, white men. Vanilla viewers are meant to come away feeling a sympathy for the vulnerability of the subjects.

Children of the Void by Regina Snow (Wildfire Club, 1997) The Wildfire Club was an independent publishing house created for the express purpose of publishing books about the all-female fantasy world Aristasia. While all of their books are quite enjoyable, the one most relevant to age play is *Children of the Void*. It follows the lives of several women and describes how they create their immersive environment. They engage in age play, school roleplay, maid training, and domestic discipline. Innocence is highly prized, but as a state of mind rather than as a lack of experience.

In a world where most fetish materials are usually aimed exclusively at men, I highly recommend this rare book to women age players.

Other Wildfire Club books which may be enjoyable include *The District Governess*, also by Regina Snow. Published in 1996, *Governess* is a collection of vignettes in Aristasia.

The last Aristasian novel that I recommend to age players, specifically those interested in corporal punishment, is *The Female Disciplinary Manual: a Complete Encyclopedia of the Correction of the Fair Sex* by the fictitious Standing Committee on Female Education. *The Manual*, which takes itself very seriously, is a simulated guide set in 2035. It instructs teachers and other educational staff on how to employ discipline in institutional settings. Descriptions of punishments and their uses are extremely detailed. This book makes a wonderful gift for Bigs who are new to domestic discipline and who might enjoy an educational experience that is also roleplay.

"Psychosexual Infantilism in Adults: the eroticization of regression" by Dr. Thomas John Speaker (Columbia Pacific University, 1986) This unpublished dissertation starts off discussing psychosexual infantilism and other issues with cognitive and sexual development. However, it does eventually begin to address actual age play, candidly discussing a number of cases and the slow, but steady development of the community. The dissertation is available at understanding.infantilism.org.

"Still in Diapers" by Tristan Taormino. (*The Village Voice*, 14 August 2002) Well-known sexuality author, activist, and educator Tristan Taormino took it upon herself to attend an ABDL party. The event was hosted by the now-defunct Still in Diapers New York, which organized through sidny.org. Her piece is sensitive and introductory in nature, explaining terms and recounting the appeal of wearing diapers and age playing. While Taormino admits that she doesn't understand the desire to engage in ABDL play, she proves to be very open-minded and even wore a diaper while writing the piece!

Community

abdlpixel.com This ABDL social media site allows members to post various media, from music to stories, and to connect with one another via groups and forums.

abdlscandinavia.com This multilanguage, inclusive site allows people to date, socialize, and post media. If you do some fishing, older pages have some educational material.

abdlstoryforum.info On this site, you can post ABDL stories, but room is also made for off-topic discussions.

adisc.org Indesputably one of the best ABDL forums online, the Adult babies, Diaper lovers, and Incontinents Support Community provides a safe space for people to talk and connect. While the forums are for adults only, they allow no explicit adult content.

dailydiapers.com This long-running social media site boasts a lot of activity, which they encourage with contests and frequent updates.

ddlgforum.com This newer forum is fast becoming a hub of community activity, run by and for the next generation. Moderators are not afraid to tweak rules as issues arise. A healthy community is nurtured and growing pains are taken in stride.

ddlgworld.com There is a lot of overlap between DDlg Forum and DDlg World. Time will tell which forum shall prevail. DDlg World seems to be a bit more kink-friendly and focused on education. There are special sub-forums dedicated to ABDL, BDSM, and pet play.

littlesmunch.com This is a great place to get started in finding your local age play community and participating in real world events.

littlespaceonline.com This forum is by and for the newer generation of age players. They host a Littles movie night where Littles can all watch a movie together and chat online.

Education

Most educational material generated by the Littles community, as opposed to the earlier infantilism and adult baby communities, is being posted to forums or social media sites like fetlife.com. This can make it a little harder to catalogue, but it also turns upkeep into a communal effort, taking the pressure off of individuals who often cease posting and updating over time. However, there are still a few sites that run independently.

adriansurley.com Adrian Surley is an incontinnent woman who dabbles in age play in the wearing of onesies and printed diapers. Her site is a mixture of a personal blog, diaper product reviews, anonymous pictures, and more. The practical updates to her blog on subjects from visiting the doctor while diapered to diaper rash treatments for adults are why her website is listed as educational.

biglittlepodcast.com The Big Little Podcast has probably done more for the Littles community in recent years than any other single entity. Hosted by Mae, Mako Allen, and Spacey, the podcast interviews age players of all kinds, discusses topics related to age play, and promoted community and personal projects.

domsub.life This static DD/lg blog was written by a DD/lg couple and takes a very gentle approach. It consists of articles offering advice and practical suggestions for new Daddy-Little relationships.

liljennie.com Started in 1994, Lil Jennie is a personal site that includes a lot of practical educational material, like definitions of infantilism and a baby talk primer. It also includes practical advice on things like being in an infantilist marriage. This site is definitely a little dated, but the information is still good!

socalab.250x.com This site provides some practical tips and hypnosis files for "un-potty training" and archives some information from Diaper Pail Friends, like their Mommy Manual. The events page seems to have been abandoned; the most recent event was from 2009.

theghidrah.com The Ghidrah is a polyamorous BDSM group made up of Mako Allen and Bob Spacey of the Big Little Podcast as well as Pene Princess. Their website lists most of their projects, including littlesmunch.com, biglittlepodcast.com, classes that they teach, and the adult baby and Littles pride symbol.

understanding.infantilism.org Painstakingly compiled by Bitter-Grey, Understanding Infantilism is still the penultimate work on infantilism and has been around since 1995. The only negative thing that I can possibly say about the site, which has been an invaluable resource to me both personally and professionally, is that it's so extensive that you can get lost in it. If you're looking for information about age play or diaper fetishsim and can't find it anywhere else, Understanding Infantilism can at least get you started and the site is constantly being improved and updated.

Movies & Television

Most average people only ever see the world of Littles on television or in movies. The following examples are useful for Littles to watch not just to learn more about ourselves, but to learn about how the world views us, how we might be treated, and which misconceptions we have yet to overcome.

Baby Doll directed by Elia Kazan (Newton Productions, 1956) This movie's infantilization of Caroll Baker's character, Baby Doll, is more about marking the difference in age between her and her husband, played by Karl Malden, than in exploring age play. That said, she is definitely infantilized. The movie is rife with age play (and blatant racism), opening by showing Baker sucking her thumb and sleeping in a child's bed, surrounded by toys. She refers to her bedroom as "the nursery" for Pete's sake. We also see the sexual tension that often results from watching adults do childish things, as when Silva Vacarro (played by Eli Wallach), suggestively rides a rocking horse. The film was released to predictable controversy and was largely banned. As a point of interest, this film resulted in the creation and popularity of the babydoll nightgown and was written by

Tennessee Williams.

Girly or *Mumsy, Nanny, Sonny, & Girly* directed by Freddie Francis (Brigitte, Fitzroy Films Ltd., Ronald J. Jahn Productions, 1970) This horror movie shows a lot of power exchange, with dominant roles being traded back and forth among the characters. The story follows New Friend, played by Michael Bryant, as he is abducted into a homicidal age play family. This movie is especially fun for Littles who are also tops or sadists and want to get fresh ideas.

The Baby directed by Ted Post (Quintet Films, 1973) This delightful horror movie (or fantasy, depending on how you look at it) is admittedly weird. It has stuck around as a sort of cult classic. It's a sort of harem show with four women all vying for control of Baby, a grown man who had been forcibly regressed by his dominant mother and two sisters.

The Phil Donahue Show (First-run Syndication, November 1991) Adult babies Ginger, Dennis, Lee, and Gene (of the Great Lakes Adult Diaper Society, or GLADS) alongside professional mommy Anne Murray and sexologist Dr. Charles Moser are featured on this program, discussing infantilism and attempting to educate the public.

The Jerry Springer Show (Syndication, October 1992) Generally regarded as the classiest of the Jerry Springer adult baby shows, this segment featured a number of guests:

- Stephanie (an ABDL)

- Tommy (of DPF)

- Heidi (William Windsor, the "baby man" of Phoenix)[3]

- Lee Carroll (adult actress and professional mommy)

- Dr. Robert R. Butterworth (psychologist)

- Dr. Mary S. Hogan (psychologist)

The show is a blend of sensitivity and shock value, with Dr. Butterworth being almost comically offended by the idea of age play. In the end, shock value won out and *The Jerry Springer Show* became what it is known for today with subsequent shows being typically raunchy and meaningless.

The Montel Williams Show (Syndication, 23 February 1992) This show again features Gene Smith, founder of GLADS, along with his partner Dee. Community founders Angela Bauer and husband Don Davis are also in attendance, along with two more ABDL men from Seattle. Dr. Jim Gordon was a last-minute replacement for the psychologist originally scheduled to appear.

A Weekend at Miss Martindale's (Channel 4, 1996) A sterling example of era age play, this British documentary follows the all-woman, roleplay environment "Aristasia", as created by Miss Marianne

Martindale. Spanking (and training someone to spank), switch roleplay, and D/s play are all charmingly depicted. For more information on Aristasia, visit aristasia-central.com, aristasia.net, or aristasia.info. There are also a number of out-of-print books about Aristasia, which are described in the pertinent section.

ER **"Dead Again"** (NBC, 3 October 2002) This was the episode that coined the term "adult baby syndrome", which was later adopted as a title for a 2003 article about an infantilist in *The American Journal of Psychiatry*. Though the appearance of the adult baby was brief, this was the first time many age players saw someone like themselves in popular media.

CSI: Crime Scene Investigation **"King Baby"** (CBS, 17 February 2005) This entire episode is dedicated to age play, albeit an over the top version of it. Due to its prime time airing, a lot of people have seen this show.

SexTV **"Submerged Beauty/Molly Crabapple/Adult Baby Nursery"** (SexTV: the Channel, 31 March 2005) This episode features photographer Polly Borland (of *The Babies*), artist and author Katherine Gates, psychotherapist Dr. Tracie O'Keefe, and a few adult babies.

The Tyra Banks Show (Syndication, 8 May 2008) A clearly uncomfortable Tyra interviews age player and diaper lover Rachel. As a result of appearing on the show, rumor has it that Rachel lost her job as a daycare worker.[4]

Secret Lives of Women "**Fetishes and Fantasies**" (WE tv, 1 April 2008) Accompanied by her face-blurred boyfriend and mother, a young woman named Kailey shares her Baby Ella persona. Ella has gone on to become a spokesperson for the age play community, appearing on the Big Little Podcast and blogging at ellasplayspace.blogspot.com. Though she seems to have stopped posting, the blog is an interesting portrayal of the daily life of a submissive age player.

Taboo "**Fantasy Lives**" (National Geographic Channel, 2 May 2011) California-based Stanley Thornton of bedwettingabdl.com and his caregiver Sandra Dias show off their nursery in this episode. After viewing the show, Republican Senator Tom Coburn of Oklahoma called for an investigation of their social security benefits. Extensive investigations showed that no fraud had been committed, but the event was still traumatizing and Stanley went through a very public suicide scare.

My Strange Addiction "**Adult Baby/Eats Dryer Sheets**" (TLC, 24 July 2011) Adult actress Riley Kilo discusses her adult baby persona, though not her adult career. Over eerie music, we hear her friend James belittle her lifestyle and ask her to "see a professional." However, upon meeting with Riley, psychotherapist Nancy Kells confirms that Riley will not abandon her Little persona. Riley also comes out as an adult baby to her friend Candice, who is visibly shaken, but ultimately supportive. Given the judgemental tones, it's surprising that the program manages to be sensitive to Riley's being transgender, mentioning it only briefly and using her proper pronouns. Riley maintains a long-running blog at staydiapered.com, where she also posts pictures and videos.

Dr. Phil "**Unusual Syndromes and Fears**" (Syndication, 18 January 2012) 24-year-old adult baby Brett and his caregiver girlfriend Cat give viewers a look into their ABDL lifestyle.

My Crazy Obsession "**Grown-Up Baby**" (TLC, 21 March 2012) After his terrible experience following his appearance on *Taboo*, it's a wonder that Stanley returned to shock television, but this time he did it on his own terms. The result was a much more realistic snapshot of his life.

The 15-Stone Babies or *I Am an Adult Baby* (Channel 4, 13 December 2012) This gentle documentary showed a number of age players, a couple of age play relationships, and some ABDL businesses. Auntie V (credited as Auntie Viv) of the now-closed Very Special Clothes made an appearance, as did Davy of toddlerism.com.

Kat Nichols of mmmdiapers.com and her partner Justin were heavily featured. Justin's employment was compromised when his boss saw the documentary. He had to move and the relationship ended as a result.[5]

Derek and Maxine of nursery-thymes.com discussed their strong marriage and struggling business, a professional nursery in England. Upon seeing the documentary, their neighbors apparently recognized them, became inebriated, and attempted to incite a brawl. The incident went to court, but the neighbors were found to be not guilty.[6]

Real Sex "**Episode 32**" (HBO, 2005) Nanny Lynette throws a birthday party for Kimmy, who is not interviewed.[7] The party includes cake, toys, professional Mommies, and lots of friends. The usual explanations take place.

Shopping

Don't forget to search for the many fine ABDL retailers on etsy.com, amazon.com, and ebay.com!

abuniverse.com AB Universe produces some of the best adult baby diapers in the business. Their diapers are thick, cute, and ever-improving. I personally recommend the space diapers--with stars that disappear when they become wet!

auntie-annie.co.uk This charming, old fashioned store focuses on sissy adult baby apparel and accessories.

awwsocute.com A newer company, Aww So Cute offers the basic range of in-house diapers (of middling quality) and clothes, but also an inflatable crib (amazing!) and baby bottle iPhone covers. Aww So Cute seems determined to corner the ABDL market and have even appeared at the Adult Video Network (AVN) Adult Entertainment Expo.

babyapparels.com Despite the name, this store has been making adult baby *furniture* since 1985.

bambinodiapers.com Bambino boasts impeccable customer service along with in-house diaper brands, including the all-white Classico, the community-favorite Bellissimo, and, my personal favorite, the Teddy. They also sell other adult diaper brands, like Molicare and Tena, and diaper boosters.

birchplaceshop.com Birch Place Shop carries feminine clothes made with sissies and crossdressers in mind. They have a special section for adult baby clothes and their selection is larger than that of many companies that specialize in Littles clothing. The quality is generally good, but they do sometimes use cheap notions, like fragile plastic snaps. Prices are generally on the high end of reasonable and everything is beautifully photographed.

cosyndry.com Cosy 'n' Dry offers a selection of adult baby and sissy clothes and accessories, including shoes which feature soft soles instead of the hard soles used in most adult shoes.

cuddlz.com Adult baby clothing, diapers, and accessories. They also offer a "waddle onesie" equipped with extra padding in the crotch area to encourage a babyish gait.

evolved-footwear.com Not actually aimed at age players, Evolved Footwear offers light-up sneakers in adult sizes.

hoverkicks.com This mainstream company also produces light-up sneakers for adults.

kunzmann.com This German site offers adult baby clothing rendered in plastic.

luckystarsleather.com Lucky Stars Leather makes a variety of premade and custom age play gear, which is also available on etsy.com. Their work is high quality and their customer service is personable and practical. Lucky Stars goes out of their way to contribute to the age play community and regularly donates items to various age play organizations.

myspecialharness.com My Special Harness offers adult-sized baby reins and bed restraints in affordable polypropylene webbing.

onesiesdownunder.com Onesies Downunder has made quite an effort to be part of the age play commuity, hiring known age players as spokesmodels and soliciting reviews for their high-quality products. Prices are affordable and they even offer gift cards!

pacifiersrus.com Pacifiers R Us offers refurbished pacifiers made from adult-size teats and cute mouth guards. You can order a premade pacifier or "build" your own.

patapoom.com This site features some of the cutest clothes and accessories for Littles available, and they're all original!

privatina.eu This German site provides beautifiul and high quality clothing and accessories for Littles in unique styles.

the-all-in-one-company.co.uk Onesies have become a bit of a fad lately and there are a number of vanilla sites that produce them, like jumpinjammerz.com and foreverlazy.com. I thought that the All-In-One Company warranted a special notice because they offer customizable onesies and feetie pajamas in precious styles.

works cited

Little Space

1. "Paraphilic infantilism." *Wikipedia: The Free Encyclopedia.* Wikimedia Foundation, Inc., 3 January 2016. Web.
2. "Dead Again." *ER.* National Broadcasting Company. 3 October 2002. Television.
3. Pate, Jennifer E. and Glen O. Gabbard. "Adult Baby Syndrome." *The American Journal of Psychiatry.* 160.11 (2003): 1932-1936. Web.
4. Money, John. *Lovemaps: Clinical Concepts of Sexual Erotic Health and Pathology, Paraphilia, and Gender Transposition in Childhood, Adolescence, and Maturity.* New York: Prometheus Books, 1986. Print.
5. "Anaclitism." *Wiktionary: A Wiki-based Open Content Dictionary.* Wikimedia Foundation, Inc., 20 November 2014. Web.

6. Stekel, Wilhelm. *Patterns of Psychosexual Infantilism*. New York: Washington Square Books, 1966. Print.

7. "List of school pranks." *Wikipedia: The Free Encyclopedia*. Wikimedia Foundation, Inc., 16 January 2016. Web.

Community

1. Rulof, Paul. *Ageplay: From Diapers to Diplomas*. Las Vegas: The Nazca Plains Corporation, 2011. Print.

2. Bauer, Angela. "Dpf Gone?" 10 December 2008. Daily Diapers Forum. Web. 20 January 2016.

3. Bittergrey. "The Birth of the ABDL Community." *Understanding Infantilism*. 29 March 2012. Web. 16 January 2016.

4. Terrynappykid's channel. "British Sex Adult Babies and sissyboys." Online video clip. *YouTube*. Google, 4 September 2009. Web. 13 October 2015. [Originally broadcast on Sky1 channel.]

5. Hausman, Eni E. "The Victorian cult of the child." *Plan Elfenbeinturm: Blog für cineastischen & literarischen Kladderadatsch*. Plan Elfenbeinturm, 10 April 2012. Web. 30 October 2015.

6. Barrie, J. M. *Peter Pan*. Project Gutenberg, 2012. *Project Gutenberg*. Web. 13 October 2015.

7. "Child Avatar." *Second Life*. Linden Research, Inc. 26 July 2015. Web. 13 October 2015.

8. United States. 108th Congress. "An Act: to Prevent Child Abduction and the Sexual Exploitation of Children, and for Other Purposes." 7 January 2003. Washington, D. C.: United States Government Publishing Office, 2003. *Library of Congress*. Web. 6 September 2015.

9. Venti, Loni. "4 Online Dating Photo Secrets From the Most-Messaged Woman on OkCupid." *Cosmopolitan*. Hearst Digital Media, 24 November 2015. Web. 4 April 2016.

10. Rudder, Christian. "The 4 Big Myths of Profile Pictures." *OkTrends: Dating Research from OkCupid*. OkCupid, 20 January 2010. Web. 30 October 2015.

11. David. "The ABDL Pride Flag." *ABDL Scandinavia*. ABDL Scandinavia, 23 October 2006. Web. 13 October 2015.

12. coy_koi, TareBear, CockyPterodactyl. "Camp Abdulia." *FetLife*. BitLove, Inc., 25 July 2012. Web. 22 September 2015.

13. Blue, Violet. "PayPal, Square and big banking's war on the sex industry: The discriminatory practice of redlining is reinvented for the 21st century." *Engadget*. AOL, Inc., 2 December 2015. Web. 2 December 2015.

14. Blue, Violet. "TinyNibbles banned by CC Bill." *TinyNibbles*. Open Source Sex, 19 December 2007. Web. 2 December 2015.

15. McAfee, Melonyce. "Adult coloring books topping bestseller lists." *CNN*. Cable News Network, 24 April 2015. Web. 6 February 2016.

16. Allen, Mako and Mae and Spacey. "Episode 103: Ageplay Coming Out Stories." Audio blog post. *The Big Little Podcast*. Big Little Podcast, 27 September 2014. Web. 26 November 2015.

17. "Babyfur." *WikiFur*. Laurence "GreenReaper" Parry, 16 January 2016. Web.

18. Barber, Penny. "Interview With Susan Wright." *International Little Miss & Mister Little*. International Little Miss & Mister Little, 22 September 2014. Web. 15 October 2015.

Scenes & Play

1. Cramer, Elizabeth. *Dom's Guide to Submissive Training: Step-by-step Blueprint on How to Train Your New Sub a Must Read for Any Dom/Master in a BDSM Relationship*. New Jersey: CreateSpace, 2013. Print.

2. Roquelaure, A. N. *The Claiming of Sleeping Beauty*. New York: Plume, 1999. Print.

Resources

1. Rosemaiden's All-Girl channel. "A Weekend at Miss Martindale's." Online video clip. *YouTube*. Google, 19 December 2006. Web. 14 November 2015. [Originally broadcast on Channel 4.]

2. "Media Tips: Interviewing on SM-Leather Fetish Issues." *NCS Freedom*. National Coalition for Sexual Freedom, 25 June 2014. Web. 13 January 2016.

3. Watson, Joe. "Baby Man." *Phoenix New Times*. 9 June 2005. Web. 2 December 2015.

4. WBDaddy. "Oh joy, another *awesome* documentary." *ABDL Story Forum*. 16 September 2011. Web. 21 September 2015.

5. Kat Nichols Channel. "Haven't Had a Daddy in a While." Online video clip. *YouTube*. Google, 14 July 2015. Web. 24 January 2016.

6. Bittergrey. "15 Stone (95 kg or 210 lb) Babies." *Understanding Infantilism*. 21 April 2013. Web. 26 January 2016.

7. cruxshadow. "Real Sex 32 - HBO." 29 October 2007. Daily Diapers Forum. Web. 24 January 2016.

ABOUT THE AUTHOR

Penny Barber is a professional Mommy, dominatrix, and switch as well as an adult actress, pornographer, phone sex operator, and sex writer. She lives in the San Francisco bay area, the age play capital of the world.

An updated list of Penny's currend projects and passions is maintained at **naughtylittleswitch.com**. If you would like to spend some time age playing with her in her nursery, visit **diaperdisciplinarian.com** for details, including rates and location. Her kinky age play, diaper fetish, and forced regression clips can be purchased for download at **pamperedpenny.com**.

Made in the USA
Las Vegas, NV
03 January 2022

40216444R00128